MARGARET ROBERTS HERB SERIES

HERBS FOR HEALING

GW00721712

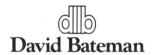

David Bateman

© Margaret Roberts 1989

Originally published by Jonathan Ball Publishers.
This edition published in 1990 by David Bateman Ltd,
'Golden Heights', 32–34 View Road, Glenfield,
Auckland 10, New Zealand

Reprinted 1992

ISBN 1 86953 021 7

A David Bateman book
Printed in Hong Kong by Colorcraft

Contents

Introduction

It was not so very long ago that most households were equipped with a large and interesting store of homemade medicines or remedies for all sorts of ailments. Grandparents taught the younger members of the family to recognise healing plants, and to make brews and decoctions, salves and lotions, until they too became proficient in home doctoring.

Doctors and apothecaries in those bygone days had only plants from which to draw their medicines, and their textbooks contained much information on the use of plants for proven prescription medicines and endless recipes for treatments using barks, berries, leaves, roots and flowers of various plants.

With the advance of twentieth century technology, the old remedies were gradually discarded and, with the improvement of medical science, families exchanged generations of folk remedies and home first aid for the new technology and synthetic medicines.

Home-grown fruit and vegetables were the exception rather than the rule and modern man's diet began largely to consist of soft, processed, hormone-injected, stabilised, flavoured and refined foods. People may well have started living longer, but whether they felt or looked better was debatable. And stress became a daily companion.

To some extent, however, today the pendulum is again swinging back to a more natural way of life. At last people are beginning to seek 'whole health'. Fresh, organically grown, unsprayed, unfertilised produce is coming into vogue once more. The refined, long-shelf-life foods are no longer as popular, and people are turning again to the home vegetable patch and herb garden for their daily needs.

Finally, therefore, those long-forgotten herbal medicines are back in demand, too, and this is what this little book is about – herbal medicines for common ailments. One of the reasons for writing it is the cries for help from the very many people who write to me. "I've tried every patent medicine. Help me, I can't go on," is a phrase I hear again and again. I know. I've been there, and I also know the deep joy of using our green heritage to soothe those common illnesses and complaints and gradually bring one to the 'high-level wellness' – the umbrella phrase for my life's work with plants.

In these pages I share with you many years of easy, healthy home treatments. I have used them on myself and on my family, and have been able to help a great many conditions. However, this is not to say that there is no place for the family doctor and I urge you to be guided by him or her at the same time. Regular medical check-ups are important. Never treat yourself or anyone else before discussing the symptoms with your doctor, and unless you are absolutely sure of the ailment and that you have identified the plant correctly. Always use your doctor, homeopath or qualified herbalist as your guide.

If you are suffering from any serious illness whatsoever – heart problems, kidney or blood conditions, chronic illnesses included – or if you are pregnant, do not try even a weak dosage of these treatments without consulting your doctor.

Herbs can act differently on different people. They also vary, in strength, flavour and size, from garden to garden. Because no single herb is a panacea, I suggest you work with one herb at a time, as I did in the beginning, and really get to know its uses and its strengths. Always test the herb first before plunging into full treatment with it. Remember that when you have read this book, you are by no means a herbalist – rather think of yourself as a pathfinder in a world of utmost satisfaction.

May your path be lined with much health and happiness.

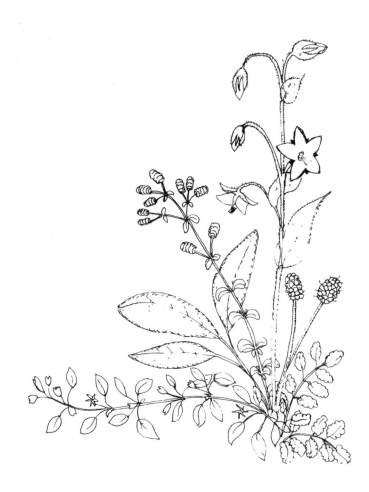

Acknowledgements

My training as a physiotherapist gave me an abiding interest in healing. To my professors and lecturers, therefore, I have a special tribute: thank you for giving me a good background which has always formed the base for my herbal healing work. Without you, I would be inadequate.

Thank you, too, to my doctor friends who have offered ideas, advice and help in working with these natural medicines. I bless you for your encouragement and assistance.

To the readers of my previous books – this book is for you, at your request, for I delight in you and your interest in herbs.

My grateful thanks go to my typist for her typing of the manuscript and to my patient editor, Alison Lowry, who makes all this possible.

Conversion Tables

Volume

mℓ to Teaspoons	mℓ to Tablespoons	mℓ to Cups	mℓ to Pints
1 mℓ = $\frac{1}{4}$ tsp	12,5 mℓ = 1 tbsp	60 mℓ = $\frac{1}{4}$ cup	570 mℓ = 1 pt
2 mℓ = $\frac{1}{2}$ tsp	25 mℓ = 2 tbsp	80 mℓ = $\frac{1}{3}$ cup	1,1 ℓ = 2 pts
5 mℓ = 1 tsp	37,5 mℓ = 3 tbsp	125 mℓ = $\frac{1}{2}$ cup	1,7 ℓ = 3 pts
10 mℓ = 2 tsp	50 mℓ = 4 tbsp	180 mℓ = $\frac{3}{4}$ cup	2,3 ℓ = 4 pts
15 mℓ = 3 tsp		250 mℓ = 1 cup	
20 mℓ = 4 tsp		500 mℓ = 2 cups	
		750 mℓ = 3 cups	
		1 litre = 4 cups	

Mass

Grams to Ounces	g/kg to Pounds
30 g = 1 oz	450 g = 1 lb
60 g = 2 oz	900 g = 2 lb
125 g = 4 oz	1,4 kg = 3 lb
250 g = 8 oz	1,8 kg = 4 lb
	2,3 kg = 5 lb

Oven Temperatures	Celsius (°C)	Fahrenheit (°F)
Very cool	100-120	210-250
Cool	130-160	270-320
Moderate	170-180	340-360
Moderately hot	190-210	370-410
Hot	220-240	430-460
Very hot	250 +	480 +

Common ailments and their treatments

Many of the following remedies are taken in the form of a herb tea. The standard brew is: 60 ml ($\frac{1}{4}$ cup) fresh herb to 250 ml (1 cup) boiling water. Stand, steep, cool for 5 minutes. Strain, then drink.

ABSCESSES AND BOILS

Cabbage   Dip a leaf in warm water and apply as a poultice to the area. Replace with a fresh leaf every now and then. Keep in place with a crêpe bandage.

Fig   Warm in the oven. Split and apply (as hot as can be tolerated). This is excellent for a boil on the gum.

Pumpkin   Roast a piece of pumpkin and apply as a poultice to the area, as hot as possible.

Onion   Apply a boiled onion, hot, to the afflicted area. When the boil bursts, wash out the area with raw onion juice diluted in water.

Castor oil plant Apply a warmed leaf as a poultice.

Radish	Slices of fresh radish can be applied to the boil and surrounding area. Hold in place with a castor oil leaf and a crêpe bandage.
Chickweed	A common weed that has wonderful drawing properties. Wash a handful in hot water, bruise slightly and apply to the area. Hold in place with a castor oil leaf or a crêpe bandage.
Honey	Honey is a strong antibiotic and wound healer. Mix with a little flour and apply to the area. Cover and keep hot (use a heating pad or hot water bottle).
Thyme	Make a strong thyme tea (125 ml thyme to 250 ml boiling water). Dip a folded clean cloth into the tea. Apply as hot as can be tolerated, then bind in place. Repeat frequently with fresh applications.

ACHES AND STRAINS (MUSCULAR) (see also SPRAINS)

Bergamot	Make a standard brew tea and drink morning and evening to soothe muscular aches and pains.
Catnip	Make a standard brew tea, adding 60 ml *Sage* and an extra 250 ml boiling water, and drink morning and evening to give relief.
Castor oil plant	Use leaf as an external application over the painful area, eg aching feet can be wrapped in warmed castor oil leaves (dip the leaves into hot water). Apply and cover with a towel and hot water bottle or heating pad.

THYME

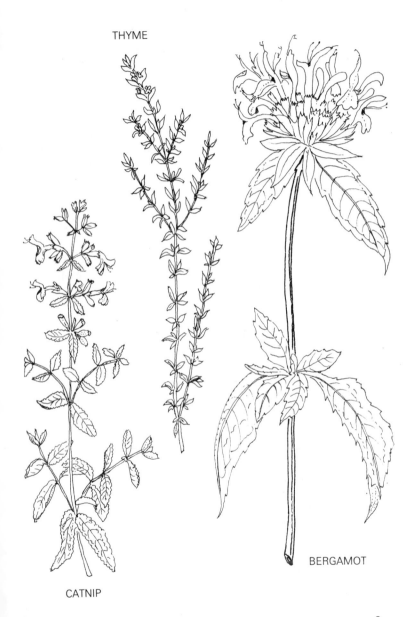

CATNIP

BERGAMOT

9

Myrtle	Make a strong brew of the leaves, using 4 cups leaves and flowers. Pour over this 1 ℓ boiling water and allow to stand and steep for an hour. Dip a cotton cloth into the tea and apply to the painful area.
Mustard	Crush a handful of mustard leaves and pour over 250 ml hot water. Apply the hot leaves to the painful area. Bind in place with a crêpe bandage. Alternatively, mix 125 ml crushed mustard seeds into a paste with 125 ml wholewheat flour and a little hot water. Add 10 ml *Apple cider vinegar*. Spread paste onto a cloth which has been wrung out in hot water and apply as hot as possible to the area. Cover or bind in place. Repeat when necessary.

See also FAVOURITE RECIPE 3: Herb tea for cramp, and 19: Herbal massage oil.

ACNE (see also SKIN DISORDERS)

Include the following in the diet: plenty of water and fresh green vegetables, especially celery, parsley, watercress, sprouts, wheat grass and sprouted wheat. Avoid fried foods, refined flour and sugar, 'junk' foods and carbonated drinks.

Elder	Make a brew of elder leaves and flowers (250 ml each) and boil up in 1 ℓ water. Use as a wash.
Rhubarb	Dry and powder the roots and mix 12,5 ml with 500 ml hot water. Dab onto the area.
Calendula	Boil up 250 ml flowers and 1 ℓ water. Cool and

10

strain, then use as a wash and lotion.

Sow's thistle   Apply the juice to the affected spot. This herb has a milky sap which dries up pimples. Apply frequently.

See also FAVOURITE RECIPE 27: Problem skin tea.

ALCOHOL ABUSE

Angelica   Make a decoction of the root by boiling up 12,5 ml root in 500 ml water. Remove from stove, stand, steep and strain. A wineglassful taken twice a day will induce a distaste for alcohol.

Cayenne   Use as a pepper on food. Alternatively, mix 25-50 ml water with 5 ml apple cider and 2 ml cayenne, and drink every evening to wean from liquor.

Chamomile   Strong chamomile tea is very soothing. Use 60 ml herb to 250 ml boiling water. Drink every night instead of alcohol.

Watercress   Eat plenty in the diet – it cleanses the liver, helps a hangover, and sweetens the breath.

Oranges   Freshly squeezed juice should be taken daily, or each time you feel like a drink. Eat whole oranges; they will help curb the desire for alcohol.

ALLERGIES

Avoid processed, refined 'white' foods, eg white flour, sugar, rice, or white of egg. Replace with extra fresh fruit and salads, oats and vegetable juices. Avoid milk and milk products while the attack is on. Drink plenty of water and avoid tea, coffee, alcohol, and carbonated drinks.

Comb honey   Chew a piece daily. This often helps clear the nose and sinuses in hayfever attacks. If possible, use the honey made in the area where you live.

Apple cider vinegar and honey drink
Mix 5-7 ml apple cider vinegar and 5-7 ml honey in a tumbler of water. Drink daily (half a glass in the morning and half in the evening).

ANAEMIA

Include the following in the diet: parsley, peas, pecan nuts, watercress, oranges, apples, apricots, barley, cabbage, cauliflower, comfrey, nettles, pumpkin, tomatoes, spinach, Brazil nuts and dandelion greens. Grated pumpkin, fresh and raw, with carrots or pineapple, is delicious. Eat grapes in season as often as possible; eat raisins when grapes are out of season.

Amaranthus   Include, fresh or cooked, in the diet.

Beetroot   Drink a wineglassful of freshly squeezed beetroot juice daily.

See also FAVOURITE RECIPE 6: Anaemia soup

ANTIBIOTIC

Natural antibiotics are: *Calendula, Garlic, Grapes, Nasturtium, Radish*, and *Thyme*. Include some of these in the diet during times of infection.

12

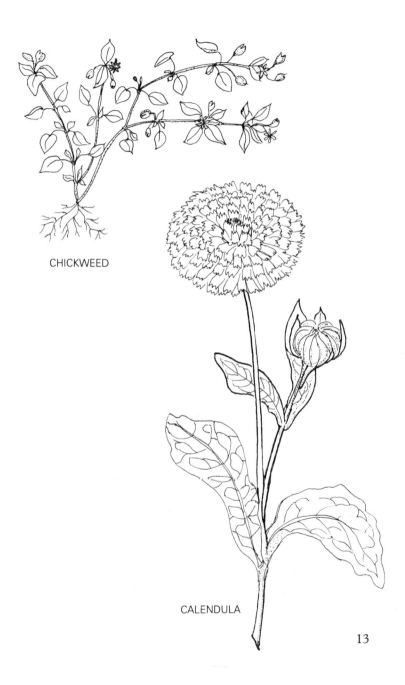

CHICKWEED

CALENDULA

13

Thyme tea
Take 60 ml fresh thyme sprigs. Pour over 250 ml boiling
water. Add a little lemon juice. Sip frequently.

ANTISEPTICS

Many plants have antiseptic properties. They can be made
into a tea or into a wash. The standard brew is 250 ml herb to
500 ml-1ℓ boiling water. Suitable herbs are: *Thyme*, *Garlic*,
Calendula, *Lavender*, *Southernwood*, *Chamomile*, *Bay*,
Myrtle, *Horseradish* and *Sage*.

ANXIETY see STRESS

ARTHRITIS

Include the following in the diet: oats, Vitamin B, celery,
comfrey, parsley, mustard, nettles, feverfew. Avoid red meat,
alcohol and starchy foods. Replace refined flours with oats, bran
and popcorn.

Comfrey Make a tea (60 ml chopped leaves to 250 ml boiling
water). Stand, steep, then drink when cool enough
to tolerate. Sweeten with honey and a little apple
cider vinegar. Drink daily.

ASTHMA (see also COUGHS)

Include the following in the diet: carrots, apples, figs, guavas,
garlic, horseradish, lemons, onions, green peppers, raisins
and oranges.

Honeysuckle Fill a bottle of honey with honeysuckle flowers, ensuring that each is
coated with honey. Eat a couple of

spoonfuls daily to ease tightness and a chesty cough.

Ginger

Boil up a thumb-length piece of root in 1 ℓ water. Sweeten with honey. Sip a little frequently.

Comfrey

Include in the diet and make into a tea, using the standard brew. Sweeten with honey if desired, and drink daily.

Verbascum (mullein)

Make tea, using flowers and young leaves. Standard brew. Sweeten with honey if desired and drink daily.

Violet

Make into a tea, using leaves and flowers. Standard brew. Sweeten with honey if desired and drink daily.

Bluegum

Pick a bunch of fresh bluegum leaves. Pour over boiling water. Make a towel tent, covering the head and bowl, and inhale the fumes.

See also FAVOURITE RECIPE 26: Herb tea for bronchitis and asthma.

ASTRINGENT

Astringent herbs check excessive external and internal secretions (eg mucous membranes, skin, etc). These herbs can be made into teas, washes, douches, enemas and lotions. *NB Do not attempt douches or enemas without consulting your doctor. Pregnant women should not attempt either.*

Herbs suitable for *external* use are: *Columbine, Catnip, Oak* bark, *Myrtle* and *Camphor* (leaves). Boil up in enough water to cover. Cool, strain, apply. Herbs suitable for *internal* use are: *Salad burnet, Violet, Verbascum, Mint* and *Marjoram*. Use 60-125 ml herb to 250 ml boiling water. Sip a cup 2-3 times a day.

BAD BREATH see HALITOSIS

BEDWETTING (see also SEDATIVE)

Here refrigerant herbs are needed, herbs which will soothe and calm; often the patient is highly strung or upset, and does not sleep well. He or she may also be plagued by nightmares.

Include the following in the diet: freshly grated carrot, celery, parsley, lemon balm (melissa), honey, lemon juice, brown rice, barley, oats, popcorn (freshly popped with a touch of sea salt). Avoid sweets, cakes, refined flours, sugars, carbonated drinks and condiments.

Catnip and marjoram tea
Take one thumb-length sprig of catnip and one thumb-length sprig of marjoram and pour over 60-125 ml boiling water. Stand, steep and strain. Sweeten with a little honey. When cool enough to drink, sip slowly just before going to sleep.

Other herbs which are effective in teas are: *Lavender, Lemon balm, Lemon verbena, Hypericum* (flowers) and *Verbascum* (mullein). Use the same standard brew.

BITES AND STINGS

Stings should be treated immediately. In the case of a bee-sting, remove the sting straightaway.

Banana   Apply the inside of the skin to the painful area.

Castor oil plant   Rub castor oil onto ticks and tickbites.

16

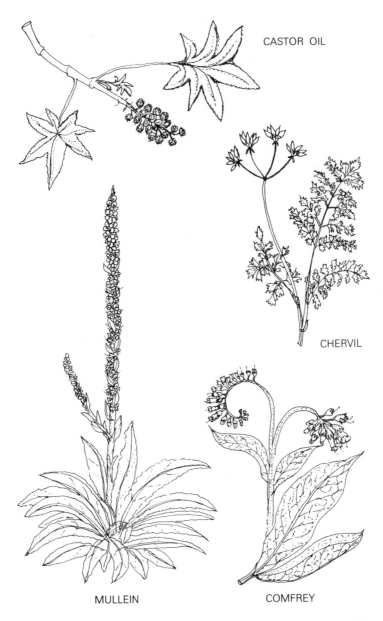

CASTOR OIL

CHERVIL

MULLEIN

COMFREY

17

Vinegar	Effective for soothing wasp stings. Dab on repeatedly.
Calendula	Squeeze the juice from the petals and apply to beestings.
Plantain	Use the leaves to rub the area. *Mint* and *Periwinkle* (Vinca rosea) are also effective.
Aloe	Split leaf open and rub the jelly onto the area.
Oats	Mix with water and apply to the area for soothing relief. (Mix with mashed banana to bring down the fever over the area.)
Onion	A slice of onion placed immediately on a beesting will draw the pain from it.
Comfrey	Squeeze the juice from the leaves to soothe a sting.
Elder	Make a strong tea of leaves and flowers and use as a wash. Dab on frequently.
Cornflower	Rub flowers into the area. *Scented geranium* leaves and flowers are good too.

BLADDER AILMENTS

Include the following in the diet: cabbage, melons (especially watermelon), mustard greens, marrows (eg gem squash, courgettes), spinach, beetroot (raw), green peppers, asparagus, orange juice (freshly squeezed), watercress and tomatoes (fresh).

Hydrangea tea
Use young leaves, 250 ml to 1 ℓ boiling water. Stand until cold. Strain. Take 2 dessertspoons at the first sign of a bladder infection. Repeat every 4 hours.

Teas can also be made using either *Parsley*, *Borage* or *Asparagus* (60-125 ml herb to 250 ml boiling water). Stand, steep, strain. Drink 3-6 times daily.

BLEEDING AND CUTS

Yarrow   Apply fresh leaves to the area.

Lemon   Apply freshly squeezed juice to the cut. Although it will sting, it will have an immediate styptic effect.

Cayenne pepper   A tiny pinch will stop bleeding from a cut. To stem internal bleeding, 2 ml in a glass of water can be effective.

Calendula   Press out the juice from the leaves and flowers and apply directly to the wound. Keep excess in the fridge as it is highly perishable.

Shepherd's purse A common weed but also an excellent styptic. Make a tea using the whole plant. Cover with boiling water, strain and, when cool enough to tolerate, use as a wash and drink the rest.

Thyme   Make a wash using 125 ml herb to 500 ml boiling water to cleanse cut.

Nettle	Make a wash as above. *Periwinkle* (Vinca major) and *Salad burnet*, using the same proportions, are also effective.
Aloe	Apply the leaf jelly to the cut.

BLOCKED NOSE see COLDS

BLOOD CLEANSER

Include the following in the diet: fresh chicory, chives, crab-apple, grapes, fresh green mustard, nettles (make a standard brew tea and add to soups and stews), sow's thistle, parsley, pumpkin and radish.

BLOOD PRESSURE

Take care to eat fresh green salads daily.

For high blood pressure include in the diet: barley, broccoli, carrots, cauliflower, celery, chives, cucumbers, endive, garlic, guavas, onions, oranges, parsley, peaches, pears, sweet peppers, purslane, pineapple, spinach, squash, strawberries, tomatoes, yarrow and cayenne pepper.

For low blood pressure include: walnuts, Brazil nuts, currants, dandelion greens, dates, figs, leeks, peas, pecan nuts, sweet potatoes, pumpkin, soya beans, raisins and pumpkin seeds.
Garlic benefits both high and low blood pressure.

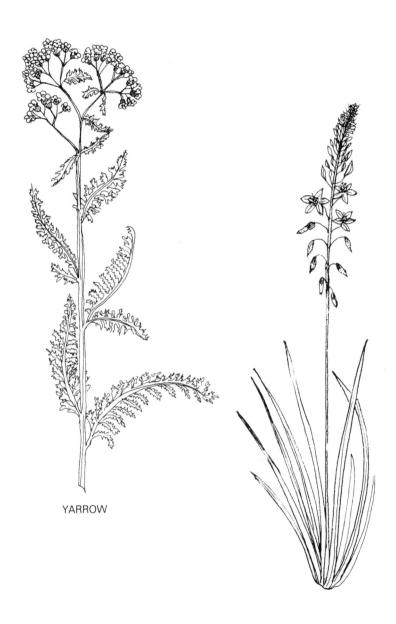

YARROW

21

Include the following in the diet: parsley, sage and celery.
Make a strong *Parsley* and *Sage* tea and use daily as a wash.

See also FAVOURITE RECIPE 21: Herb deodorant.

BOILS see ABSCESSES AND BOILS

BREASTS

Peaches   For a painful, infected breast make a strong peach leaf tea (750 ml leaves to 1,5 ℓ boiling water). Apply as a poultice several times a day.

Parsley   For hard breasts, apply bruised parsley and/or *Cabbage* leaves as a poultice. Place leaves (first warm in hot water and pat dry) inside your bra, and keep in place for 2-3 hours. Replace with fresh leaves.

Comfrey   Make a strong comfrey and yarrow tea (250 ml herb to 250 ml boiling water). Use as a wash or lotion for cracked, sore nipples. A compress worn in the bra will also bring relief (pulp root and leaf).

Carrot   Grated raw carrot can be used as a compress in the bra for sore nipples, as well as pulped leaves and juice of *Yarrow*.

Borage   For breastfeeding mothers, to promote milk flow drink a standard brew tea three times a day. *Fennel*, *Dill*, *Fenugreek* or *Parsley* tea, taken three times a day, are all effective too.

Sage   When weaning a baby from the breast, to reduce

22

milk flow drink a standard brew tea three times a day.

BRONCHITIS (see also CHEST AILMENTS and COUGHS)

Include the following in the diet: fresh asparagus, fresh grated beetroot, fresh grated carrots, cabbage, broccoli, dandelion greens, garlic, onions, chives, leeks, lettuce, pawpaw, parsley, pineapple, sweet potatoes, oranges, lemons, mandarins and watercress.

Make a strong herb tea (standard brew); any of these herbs are excellent: *Comfrey*, *Honeysuckle flowers*, *Bergamot*, *Verbascum* (mullein) or *Violets*. Drink frequently during the illness.

See also FAVOURITE RECIPE 26: Herb tea for bronchitis and asthma.

BRUISING

Cabbage	Dip leaves into hot water and bruise them by breaking the veins. Apply warmed to the painful area.
Castor oil plant	Dip leaves into hot water and bruise. Apply warmed to the area.
Comfrey	Dip leaves into hot water. Apply warmed to the area.
Marjoram	Apply a pack of warmed marjoram to the bruise. Hold in place with a crêpe bandage.
Caraway	Bruise caraway seeds in hot water and

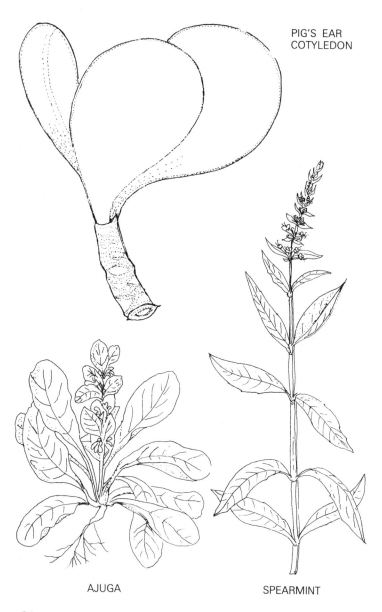

PIG'S EAR
COTYLEDON

AJUGA

SPEARMINT

24

mix into a paste with breadcrumbs. Apply hot to the bruise.

Onion   Apply slices of raw onion to the area. Bind in place.

Apple cider vinegar   Dip a cloth into either warmed or chilled apple cider vinegar and apply to the bruising. Do not use on sensitive skins or around sensitive areas (eg the eyes).

Yarrow   Dip leaves into hot water and apply to the area. Bind in place.

BURNS

Arum lily   Apply a fresh leaf to the area.

Aloe   Apply the inner, jelly-like leaf to the painful area.

Potato   Place the inner side of the peel onto the burn.

CALLOUSES AND CORNS

Ivy   Soak a leaf in vinegar and salt – 25 ml of each – overnight. The following night bind the leaf over the area and leave on for twelve hours. Repeat the procedure nightly until the area softens and peels away.

Comfrey   Chop a piece of comfrey leaf finely and squeeze out as much juice as possible. Apply juice to the area nightly. Bind in place.

Include the following in the diet: grated fresh carrots and a little chopped carrot leaves, fresh parsley, violet flowers and leaves (NB *Viola odorata*, the common garden violet), grapes (including leaves and a few tendrils) and elder flowers.

CHAPPED SKIN, HANDS

Leek	Blend leek juice into your favourite handcream. Chop leek leaves and roots finely, put through a juice extractor.
Oats	Use soaked oats as a rub or blend with liquid soap as a wash.
Comfrey	Add the juice to your favourite handcream.
Castor oil plant	Rub a little oil into the area every night.
Olive oil, almond oil	Rub a little oil into the area every night.

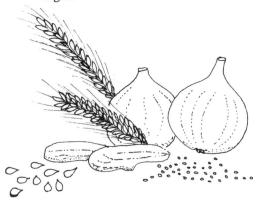

CHEST AILMENTS (see also BRONCHITIS)

Include the following in the diet: oranges, lemons, mandarins, fresh carrots, elderberries, garlic, horseradish (freshly grated root), onions, chives, parsley, green pepper, spinach and watercress.

Make a standard brew tea of any of these herbs: *Comfrey, Elder, Verbascum* (mullein), *Violet* or *Honeysuckle* (flowers).

CHILBLAINS

Include the following in the diet: dandelion greens, figs and guavas.

Cayenne pepper	Include in the diet in winter. Add *a little* to talcum powder and dust the feet before going out on a bitterly cold day. Cayenne keeps the body warm.
Ginger	Use powdered ginger as a condiment. Add to talcum powder and dust the feet.
Onion	Roast and use as a poultice on the chilblain. Bind in place. If the skin is unbroken, use a slice of raw onion on the area.
Potato	Bake and mash the inside. Mix with a little medicinal olive oil or sunflower oil. Apply warm to the area.

CIRCULATION see FAVOURITE RECIPE 13: Poor circulation herb drink.

COLD SORES see FEVER BLISTERS

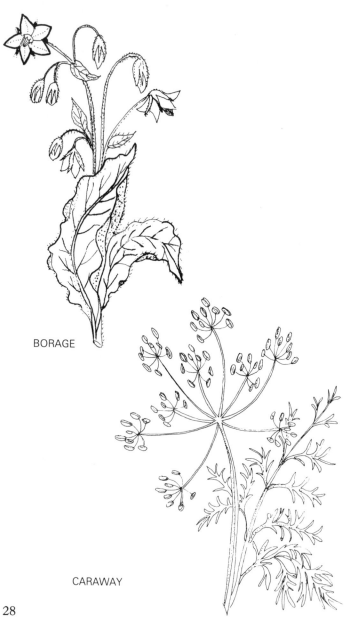

BORAGE

CARAWAY

COLDS (see also COUGHS and SORE THROAT)

Include the following in the diet: Vitamin C (500–1 000 mg daily), carrots, dandelion greens, spinach, oranges, grapefruit, guavas, horseradish (freshly grated root on bread), onions, chives, green peppers, elder flowers, elderberries, cabbage, Brussels sprouts, tomatoes, turnips and watercress.

Make a standard brew of any of these herbs: *Thyme, Sage, Lemon balm* (melissa), *Bergamot, Violet* (good for a blocked nose), *Verbascum, Elder, Lucerne, Winter savory, Borage, Peppermint* or *Yarrow*. Use as a gargle and drink at frequent intervals until the symptoms ease.

Pennyroyal	Bruise herb and inhale the strong fragrance to help clear a blocked nose.
Peppermint	Make standard brew tea and inhale fumes to clear blocked nose. *Eucalyptus* leaf tea is also effective.
Olbas	A drop on the outside of each nostril will clear a blocked nose.
Sage	Chew a fresh sage leaf (a *Nasturtium* leaf or a sprig of *Thyme* will do as well).
Cayenne pepper	Sprinkle on food and mix into teas (2 ml). It induces perspiration which brings down fever and eliminates poisons and bacteria from the body.
Garlic	Use fresh garlic in food. Chopped garlic between two slices of brown bread is excellent. Chew a sprig of parsley to freshen the breath.

Honey and lemon   Make into a hot drink with boiling water and a sprig of peppermint. Drink just before going to bed.

See also FAVOURITE RECIPE 2: Fever drink, and 12: Winter warm tonic.

CONJUNCTIVITIS (see also EYE AILMENTS)

Include the following in the diet: barley water, grated apple, asparagus, green beans, cabbage, cauliflower, dandelion greens, grapefruit, lemons, lettuce, oranges, pawpaw, parsley, prunes, spinach, sweet potatoes, wheatgerm and watercress.

Cornflowers   Make a tea using 60 ml herb to 250 ml boiling water. Use as above.

Cloves   Place 5 cloves in 250 ml boiling water. Use as above.

CONSTIPATION

Include the following in the diet: raw beetroot grated with apple, barley water, cabbage, raw and lightly steamed, grated raw carrots, celery stalks and leaves, dates, sweetcorn, pawpaw, peaches, grapes, lettuce, onions, chives, green peas, pears, fennel (leaves and stem), sprouts (mung beans and alfalfa in particular), fresh pineapple, pumpkin seeds, raw spinach leaves, quince, radish, raisins, rhubarb, sesame seeds, soya beans, squash, turnips, fresh tomatoes, fresh strawberries, walnuts and bran.

Violets Make a strong tea (125 ml leaves and flowers to 250 ml boiling water). Sweeten with honey and drink first thing in the morning.

Prunes Soak overnight in water and eat first thing each morning. *Figs*, fresh or dried, soaked overnight in water are also effective.

Honey Replace sugar with honey in your diet.

Apple Eat an apple first thing in the morning.

CONVULSIONS

Include the following in the diet: brown rice and cabbage (lightly steamed).

Make a standard brew tea from *Fennel, Catnip* or *Chamomile*. Drink a little at intervals during the day.

CORNS see CALLOUSES AND CORNS

COUGHS (see also BRONCHITIS, ASTHMA, COLDS AND SORE THROAT)

Include the following in the diet: apricots, asparagus, green beans, beetroot and beetroot tops, broccoli, cabbage, carrots, dandelion greens, lettuce, mustard, oranges, lemons, mandarins, grapefruit, parsley, peaches, pawpaw, peas, pecan nuts, watercress, spinach and garlic.

Make a standard brew tea using either *Lemon balm, Sage, Elder flowers, Honeysuckle, Verbascum* (mullein), *Thyme, Comfrey* or *Peppermint*, and drink throughout the day.

Almonds Grind 6 almonds into a meal, add 250 ml warm

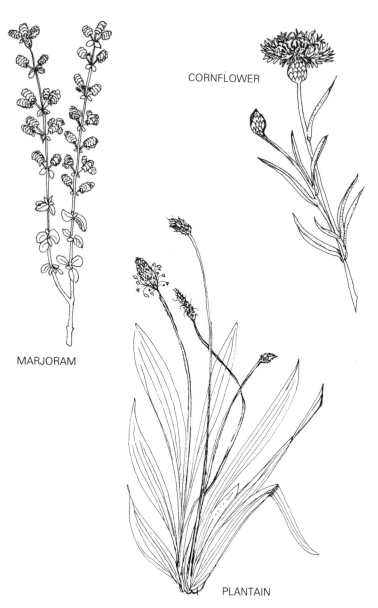

CORNFLOWER

MARJORAM

PLANTAIN

water and the juice of one lemon. Sweeten with honey. Drink a little every now and then to break the cough.

Anise   Crush 12,5 ml aniseed, then pour over 250 ml boiling water. Sweeten with honey. Allow to stand overnight. Drink a spoonful at regular intervals to soothe the cough.

Sage   Finely chop 25-50 ml fresh sage. Add enough honey to bind it (about 25 ml). Add 12,5 ml lemon juice and mix well. Keep near at hand and take a teaspoon each time you cough.

Onion   Cut onion into thin slices, sprinkle each slice with sugar and cover. Leave overnight. Drain off the juice and take a teaspoon every now and then to relieve the cough.

See also FAVOURITE RECIPE 11: Elderflower gargle, and 12: Winter warm tonic.

CRAMPS AND MUSCLE SPASMS (see also ACHES AND STRAINS)

Make a standard brew tea using either *Chamomile*, *Rosemary*, *Ginger*, *Peppermint* or *Apple cider vinegar*. Add honey to sweeten. Take 5 ml daily in a glass of water to ease cramps.
    Calcium tablets (Dolomite) and Vitamin C (500 g daily) will also ease cramp.

Eucalyptus Rub oil (or *Apple cider vinegar*) into the painful area.

See also FAVOURITE RECIPE 3: Herb tea for cramp.

CUTS see BLEEDING AND CUTS

CYSTITIS

Include the following in the diet: fresh (or tinned) asparagus, celery, borage, lettuce, parsley, pawpaw, watermelon, honeydew melon and barley water (drink the water and eat the barley with only herb seasoning, eg thyme, celery seeds).

Make a tea (125 ml herb to 500 ml boiling water) using either *Celery*, *Borage* or *Parsley*. Stand, then strain. Drink warm (6-12 cups per day).

Garlic tea
Crush 2-3 cloves garlic and pour over 250 ml boiling water and 12,5 ml lemon juice. Drink 4 cups of this tea at intervals throughout the day. Chew a sprig of parsley afterwards to cleanse the breath.

DEODORANT

Include sage and parsley in the diet. Chew cloves, cumin and cinnamon.

Sage   Make a tea, using 60 ml chopped sage to 250 ml boiling water. Add 3 cumin seeds and/or 5 ml broken cinnamon pieces and/or 5 cloves. Drink a cup daily.

Sage and parsley wash
Place 250 ml sage and 250 ml parsley in a saucepan. Pour over 500-750 ml boiling water and boil up for 3 minutes. Remove from heat. Stand and strain off when cool. Use as a wash daily. Keep excess in the fridge.

DEPRESSION see STRESS

After over-indulgence of alcohol, incorrect eating, smoking, or in times of anger, stress and anxiety, the following herbs will help rid the body of harmful toxins.

Include the following in the diet: celery, parsley, sage, salad burnet, fennel, thyme, rosemary, watercress, radishes, beet-root, melons (particularly watermelon), sunflower seeds, sesame seeds and apple cider vinegar.

Cayenne pepper	Take small pinches of cayenne pepper in a glass of water. Add 5-10 ml apple cider vinegar.
Fennel	Make a tea (4 cups leaves, flowers and seeds in 2 ℓ boiling water). Stand, steep, strain. Drink 1 cup and use the rest as a wash or pour in with your bathwater.
Peaches	Boil 10 peach pips in 1,5 ℓ water for 10 minutes. Cool, strain and keep in the fridge. Take 12,5 ml four times a day to cleanse the system. (This is especially good for treating worms.)
Sea salt	Add 250-500 ml to your bathwater and soak in the bath for half an hour. Rub a handful of salt into the feet. After an X-ray add 500 ml sea salt, 250 ml bicarbonate of soda and 500 ml Epsom salts to the bathwater to offset the effects of radiation.

Sweet basil and clove tea
Take 60 ml basil and 6 cloves. Pour over 250 ml boiling water. Stand, steep, strain. Drink while hot.

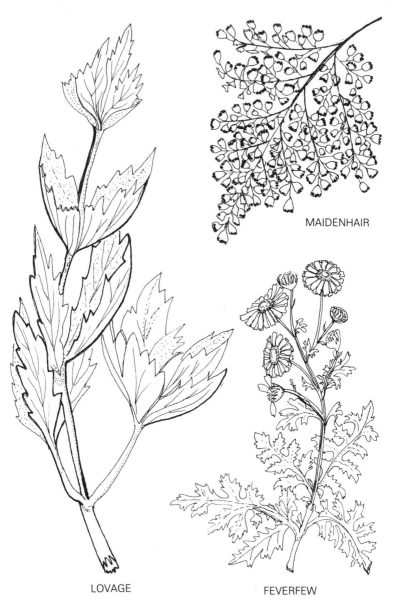

MAIDENHAIR

LOVAGE

FEVERFEW

36

DIABETES

Include the following in the diet: prickly pears, green vegetables, sunflower seeds, cabbage, celery, olives, parsley, soya beans and mandarins.

Make a standard brew tea of *Nettle*. Drink daily.

DIARRHOEA

Include the following in the diet: white rice, barley water, grated apple, grated quince, cream crackers and flat Coca-Cola.

Make a standard brew tea using either *Scented geranium*, *Ginger* root, *Yarrow*, *Peppermint*, *Periwinkle* (Vinca major, *Waterlily* or *Amaranthus*.

DIURESIS

Include the following in the diet: grapes, apples, melons (particularly watermelon), raw onions, asparagus, celery, parsley, pawpaw and strawberries.

Make a standard brew tea using either *Fennel*, *Celery*, *Nettle*, *Yarrow*, *Sweetcorn* husk silk or *Parsley*.

DIZZINESS

Include the following in the diet: fresh fruit juices, vegetables juices, beetroot, cabbage, carrots, barley, sweetcorn, mushrooms, onions, green peas, baked potatoes, soya beans, sunflower seeds and turnips.

Make a standard brew tea using either *Rosemary*, *Mint* or *Lemon balm* (melissa) to combat dizzy spells.

Include the following in the diet: beetroot and fresh coconut.

Make a standard brew tea using either *Scented geranium, Ginger, Hypericum, Quince, Yarrow* or *Peppermint.* Drink frequently.

Include the following in the diet: grated fresh carrots, lettuce, dandelion greens, salad burnet, chickweed, pawpaw, parsley, peaches, sweet potatoes, green peas, pecan nuts, prunes, watercress and spinach.

NB Consult your doctor before attempting to treat earache, and particularly ear infections in children.

Caraway Crush 125 ml seeds. Heat a slice of bread in the oven and discard crusts. Pound seeds and bread together. Add a little hot brandy. Apply as a poultice behind the ear.

Garlic Peel 2-3 cloves, encase in a piece of gauze and insert gently into the extreme outer canal of the ear. *Do not push too far in.*

Verbascum Oil can be bought from a chemist or homeopathic supplier. Use a warmed drop or two in the ear, or apply a poultice of warmed flowers to the outer ear or behind it.

Onion Apply a roast onion, as hot as can be tolerated, to the area behind the ear.

Yarrow Make a strong tea (125 ml herb to 250 ml boiling water). Dip a ball of cottonwool in the tea, wring

out and apply behind the ear, or insert (not too
deeply) into the ear.

Include the following in the diet: sprouts (especially mung
beans and alfalfa), apricots, dried beans, lentils, fresh grated
beetroot, Brazil nuts, broccoli, carrots, cauliflower, cabbage,
sweetcorn, sesame seeds, sunflower seeds, guavas, horseradish,
lemons, lettuce, mustard greens, oranges, parsley, peaches, peçan
nuts, green peppers, sweet potatoes, honey, soya beans, spinach,
tomatoes and watercress.

Make a standard brew tea using *Salad burnet*, *Calendula*
(leaves and flowers), *Lavender* or *Nettle*. Drink daily.

Aloe   Apply the leaf jelly to the affected area.

Strawberries Pulp fresh strawberries and apply to the area.

Grapes   Pulp the flesh of the grapes and apply to the
                area.

Oatmeal   Mix with water and apply to the area.

Elder   Make a wash (250 ml flowers and leaves to 750
                ml boiling water). Stand and steep. Strain
                when the wash is quite cool. Dab on fre-
                quently. Store excess in the fridge. A wash
                using the same proportions can be made from
                Nettle, *Ajuga*, *Calendula*, *Grape leaves* and
                Soapwort (Saponaria officinalis).

Burdock   The leaves can be used to make a wash (250 ml

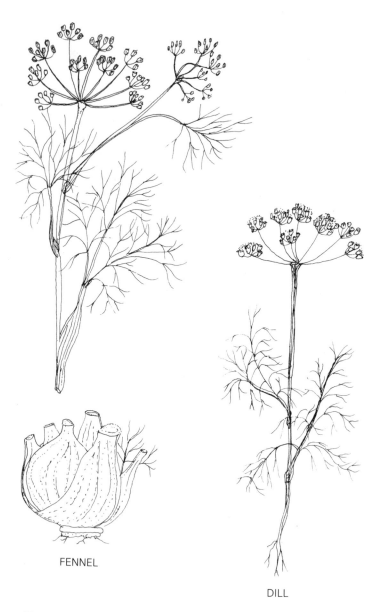

FENNEL

DILL

leaves to 750 ml boiling water) and lotion. They are an excellent treatment for many skin conditions, especially eczema. The leaves can be eaten as a vegetable.

Soapwort   Chop roots, leaves and flowers, cover with water and boil for 15 minutes. Leave to cool. Makes a soapy, green, soothing wash and lotion. Dab on frequently. Keep excess in the fridge. Excellent for scalp eczema; use as a shampoo.

EYE AILMENTS (see also CONJUNCTIVITIS)

Include the following in the diet to improve eyesight, clear infections and generally strengthen the eyes: borage, calendula, apples, raw beetroot (including leaves), broccoli, carrot, cabbage, coconut, watercress, strawberries, watermelon, grapefruit, lemons, lettuce, onions, nasturtiums, prunes, chicory, grapes, sesame seeds and sunflower seeds.

Cucumber   For tired eyes, place fresh slices over the lids and rest for half an hour.

Cabbage   Boil 250 ml chopped leaves in 1 ℓ water. Use the water as a wash.

Fennel   Chop up 12,5 ml herb. Pour over 250 ml boiling water. Dip a clean cloth into the tea and use as a compress. *Thyme, Cornflower* and *Yarrow* can all be used in the same way.

FAINTING

Include the following in the diet: barley (as a drink and eaten

cooked), sunflower seeds, Brazil nuts, pecan nuts and walnuts.

Make a standard brew tea using either *Rosemary* or
Lucerne.

FEVER

Include the following in the diet: barley water (add a pinch of
cayenne pepper), grapes, diluted grape juice.

Drink as much cool water as possible; hold ice chips be-
tween the lips.

Make a standard brew tea of *Borage*, *Catnip*, *Yarrow* or
Tansy.

Lemons   Suck slices of ice-cold lemon.

Brown rice   Cook 250 ml rice in 1,5 ℓ water. Allow to cool,
                then strain and drink the water.

Strawberries Liquidise with cool water and drink. (To 125
                ml berries add a few *Borage* flowers and 2
                leaves in 250 ml water. Liquidise.)

See also FAVOURITE RECIPE 2: Fever drink

FEVER BLISTERS

Apply leaf jelly of *aloe* frequently, or dab on *Apple cider
vinegar*.

FLATULENCE

Include the following in the diet: asparagus, grated fresh beetroot, endive, mustard, peaches, tomatoes, and olives.

Make a standard brew tea using either *Mint* (particularly
Peppermint), *Bergamot*, *Catnip*, *Lemon verbena* or *Tarragon*.

Anise   Chew a few aniseeds (or *Caraway* seeds).

See also FAVOURITE RECIPE 7: Herb tea for stomachache.

FRACTURES

Comfrey   Make a standard brew tea and drink three times a day. Include comfrey daily in the diet. Pulp the comfrey leaf and piece of root and pour hot water over it. Spread the mixture onto a bandage and bind in place over the area.

Sesame seeds Include sesame seeds in your daily diet. *Sunflower seeds* can also be included.

Calcium   Take 2-3 bone flour and dolomite tablets daily to strengthen and help bones knit.

GALLBLADDER DISORDERS see FAVOURITE RECIPE 8: Liver and gallbladder tonic.

GLANDS

Include the following in the diet: oats, broccoli, kelp, artichoke, melons, pears, apples and Vitamin C.

Apple cider vinegar To reduce glandular swellings, dip a clean cloth in apple cider vinegar and apply to the area as a compress. Keep it warm and covered.

Burdock   Bruise a leaf and warm it in hot water. Apply to the area.

Cumin   Soak 250 ml cumin seeds in brandy

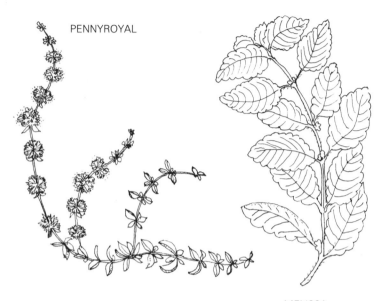

PENNYROYAL

MELISSA

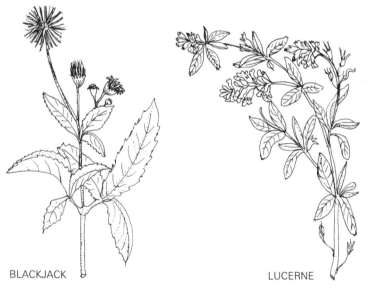

BLACKJACK

LUCERNE

44

	overnight. Apply to the area and bind in place.
Fennel	Apply fennel leaves, warmed and bruised, to swollen glands.
Hydrangea	Make a compress of leaves, warmed and bruised, and apply to the area. *Ivy* leaves can be used in the same way (externally only).

GOUT

Include the following in the diet: cabbage, carrots, celery, cucumbers, grapes, lettuce, fresh sliced mushrooms, parsley, figs, strawberries, tomatoes, cauliflower and grated, fresh, raw beetroot, nettles and asparagus.

Make a standard brew tea using either *Parsley*, *Rosemary* or *Sage* and drink daily.

Sage   Make a strong sage tea and apply as a compress.

Comfrey   Mash and pulp the leaf and root and apply as a compress.

See also FAVOURITE RECIPE 1: Rheumatism tea.

GRAZES

Make a strong brew (125 ml herb to 250 ml boiling water) from *Rosemary*, *Salad burnet*, *Thyme* or *Yarrow* and use as a wash.

Aloe   Apply jelly from leaf to the grazed area. *Waterlily* (stem and leaf) are also soothing.

Include the following in the diet: broccoli, Brussels sprouts, guavas, grapefruit, horseradish (freshly grated root on bread), lemons, oranges, parsley, green peppers, spinach, tomatoes, watercress, and nasturtium leaves.

For all mouth problems, make a strong tea using either *Sage*, *Thyme*, *Oregano*, *Comfrey*, *Lucerne* or *Carrot* leaves. Use to gargle or dab onto sore gums.

Apple cider vinegar	Dilute and rinse the mouth out with the liquid.
Peaches	Boil up 8 peach pips in 1 ℓ water for 20 minutes. Using small quantities, rinse the mouth out several times a day.

HAEMORRHAGE

Include the following in the diet: comfrey, sunflower seeds, parsley, bananas, cayenne pepper and lemons.

Yarrow Bruise leaves and scald with hot water. Apply as a local compress. Alternatively, make a standard brew tea, dip a clean cloth into it and apply. The same tea can be used as a drink – sip frequently until the bleeding stops. *Nettle* tea can be used in the same way.

HAEMORRHOIDS

Include the following in the diet: sweet potatoes bananas, beans, plums, sweetcorn, prunes and pumpkin.

Comfrey   Pulp leaves and roots and apply as a compress.
           Pulp *Yarrow* leaves and use in the same way.

Myrtle   Make a strong tea (60-125 ml herb to 250 ml boil-
           ing water). Stand, steep, strain and use as a wash.
           Yarrow, *Scented geranium* and *Thyme* tea can be
           used in the same way.

HAIR

Include the following in the diet: apples, apricots, asparagus, raw grated beetroot, carrots, broccoli, cabbage, coconuts (flesh and milk), dandelion, chickweed, sow's thistle, oats, lemons, lettuce, onions, prunes, radishes, brown rice, summer squash, watercress and turnips.

To stimulate growth and ensure good condition, and to keep the scalp dandruff free, brew strong teas of the following herbs: *Rosemary*, *Sage*, *Sweet basil*, *Bergamot*, *Maidenhair fern*, *Quince* (skins, cores and a few leaves), *Chamomile*, *Soapwort* or *Pink Australian phlox* (Saponaria officinalis), *Nettle*, *Burdock* and *Rhubarb* leaf. For fair hair: use chamomile and rhubarb leaf; for dark hair use rosemary and sage. Boil up a potful of herb with enough water to cover. Boil for 5 minutes, then stand and cool. Strain and use either as a rinse or massage into the scalp.

HALITOSIS

Include the following in the diet: peas, potatoes, brown rice, comfrey, and barley.

Chew *Mint*, *Thyme*, *Rosemary*, *Sage* or *Parsley* to freshen the breath.

Gargle with strong *Sage*, *Rosemary* or *Thyme* tea.

See also FAVOURITE RECIPE 28: Herbal mouthwash.

47

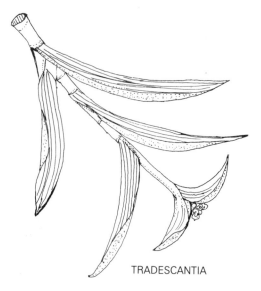

TRADESCANTIA

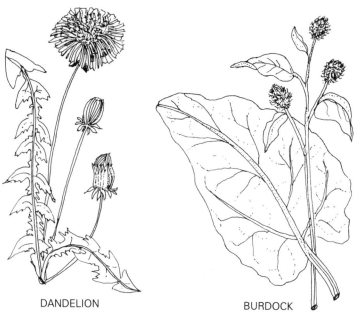

DANDELION

BURDOCK

Include the following in the diet: apples, barley, carrots, fresh raw grated beetroot, celery, cauliflower, figs, garlic, guavas, lemons, horseradish, onions, oranges, peaches, green peppers, raisins, mandarins, turnips and dandelion greens. Avoid all refined foods, carbonated drinks and wheat products, and use milk products with caution.

Make a standard brew tea using either *Violet* (leaves and flowers), *Mint* (particularly *Peppermint*), *Lucerne*, *Thyme* or *Lavender*.

Eucalyptus	Make a strong brew of the leaves. Place a towel tent over the head and bowl and inhale. *Lavender* leaves and flowers, *Pennyroyal* and *Pine* needles also make effective inhalants.
Olbas	A drop dabbed onto the nostrils, or a few drops in hot water, used as above, will relieve symptoms.

See also FAVOURITE RECIPE 25: Hayfever tea.

HEADACHES

Include the following in the diet: barley water, green beans, fresh raw grated beetroot, fresh raw grated carrots, walnuts, almonds, sweetcorn, lettuce, garlic, green peas, comfrey, brown rice, tomatoes and lemon juice in water. Avoid all alcohol, refined foods and sugars.

Make a standard brew tea using either *Feverfew, Lavender, Violet* (leaves and flowers), *Mint* (particularly *Peppermint*), *Rosemary, Lemon balm* (melissa), *Sweet basil, Marjoram* or *Sage*.

Calcium	Increase intake of calcium in the diet.

| *Apple cider vinegar* | Dilute 10 ml in a glass of water and sip a little every day. |

See also FAVOURITE RECIPE 4: Headache tea.

HEART CONDITIONS

Any suspected heart condition must be reported to your doctor at once.

Include the following in the diet: onions, garlic, chives, spring onions, lemons, asparagus, barley (drink the water and eat cooked grains), walnuts, pecan nuts, soya beans, and green peas.

Make a standard brew tea of either *Yarrow* or *Rosemary* and drink regularly.

HEARTBURN (see also INDIGESTION)

| *Mint* | Chew a leaf for speedy relief. |

| *Fennel* | Chew a piece of leaf or make a standard brew tea. *Lavender* and *Lemon verbena* are also effective as teas. |

| *Anise* | Chew a few *Anise* seeds or *Caraway* seeds. |

| *Peppermint* | A standard brew tea is excellent after a heavy meal. |

See also FAVOURITE RECIPE 15: Herb tea digestive aid.

HYSTERIA see FAVOURITE RECIPE 22: Herb tea for shock.

INDIGESTION (see also HEARTBURN)

Include the following in the diet: passion fruit, chicory, gooseberries, barley, green beans, raw grated beetroot, carrots, cu-

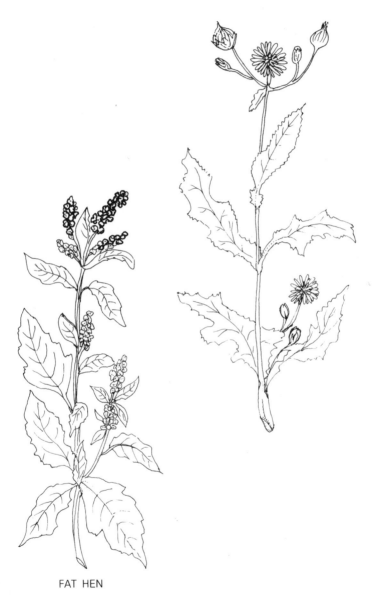

FAT HEN

cumbers, peas, baked potatoes, pumpkin, brown rice, spinach, strawberries, turnips, tomatoes, sunflower seeds, almonds, crab-apple and apple cider vinegar.

Make a standard brew tea using *Rosemary, Oregano, Lavender, Mint* (especially *Peppermint*), *Hyssop, Lemon verbena, Lemon thyme, Lovage, Catnip, Chamomile, Dill* and *Fennel*.

Caraway	Chew a few seeds to relieve indigestion. *Fennel* seeds, *Aniseed* and *Coriander* seeds are also soothing.

See also FAVOURITE RECIPE 15: Herb tea digestive aid.

INFLAMMATION, INFECTIONS

Include the following in the diet: plenty of lemon juice, broccoli, Brussels sprouts, cauliflower, endive, grapefruit, oranges, lemons, guavas, horseradish, parsley, green peppers, spinach, tomatoes, turnips and watercress.

Make a standard brew tea using *Comfrey, Thyme, Catnip, Marjoram* or *Salad burnet*.

Mustard	Mix mustard powder with a little oatmeal and hot water and use as a compress or poultice.
Comfrey	Mince the leaf and root and apply as a compress.
Apple cider vinegar	Dip a clean cloth into the vinegar, wring out and apply, frequently, to the area.

Cabbage	Bruise a leaf, warm in hot water and apply to the area. Bind in place.

See also FAVOURITE RECIPE 5: Herb tea for pain and inflammation.

INFLUENZA

Include the following in the diet: plenty of lemon juice, fresh unsweetened orange juice, alfalfa (lucerne) sprouts, leeks, onions, garlic, parsley, melons (mashed), pawpaw, grated apple and plain yoghurt.

Make a standard brew tea using either *Lemon grass, Lemon verbena, Lemon thyme, Sage, Thyme, Comfrey, Winter savory* or *Lucerne.*

See also FAVOURITE RECIPE 2: Fever drinks, and 18: Vinegar of the Four Thieves.

INSECT BITES see BITES AND STINGS

INSECT REPELLENT

To keep insects at bay and avoid bites and stings, burn any of these herbs: dried *Rosemary, Thyme, Southernwood, Sweet basil, Rue, Santolina, Tansy, Mint, Lavender* or *Pennyroyal.* You can rub pennyroyal onto the skin too, as well as sweet basil, mint and lavender. Check on the inside of the arm first for a skin reaction.

Make a strong brew to use as a lotion or wash of *Elder, Camphor, Myrtle, Mint, Lavender* or *Sweet basil.* Pick a potful of herb, cover with water and bring to the boil. Boil for 5 minutes, then stand, steep, cool and strain. Dab on frequently. Keep excess in the fridge. A particularly effective combination is lavender and elder.

To keep ants away from the home, sprinkle the following

into antholes, in bookcases and in cupboards: *Tansy, Southernwood, Rue* or *Santolina*.

To get rid of silverfish, use *Southernwood.* Place behind books, in cupboards and under carpets.

INSOMNIA

Include the following in the diet: apples, avocado, barley, walnuts, almonds, cabbage, celery, sweetcorn, leeks, lettuce, endive, fresh sliced mushrooms, onions, spring onions, green peas, baked potatoes, brown rice, soya beans, spinach, turnips and tomatoes.

Make a standard brew tea using *Lavender, Lemon balm* (melissa), *Chamomile, Catnip, Elderflower, Ginger* (root) or *Rose* petals.

Lavender   Make a 'peace pillow' by stuffing a pillow with dried leaves and flowers. *Lemon verbena* and *scented geranium* leaves also work wonders.

See also FAVOURITE RECIPE 16: Herb tea sleep aid.

IRRITABILITY (see also STRESS, NERVOUS TENSION and SEDATIVE)

Include the following in the diet: barley, almonds, peas, lentils, bran, brown rice, honey, sweetcorn, rye, sesame seeds, sunflower seeds, soya beans, lettuce, mushrooms, watercress and potatoes.

Make a standard brew tea using either *Lemon balm* (melissa), *Comfrey, Borage*, or *Lucerne*. Add 2–8 cloves to these teas and sip at intervals, throughout periods of tension.

ITCHING

Aloe   Rub the irritation with the leaf jelly to relieve itching. Burdock leaves will also give relief.

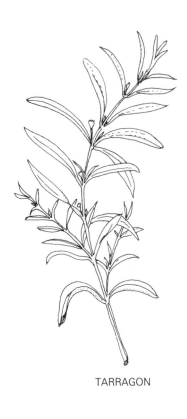

TARRAGON

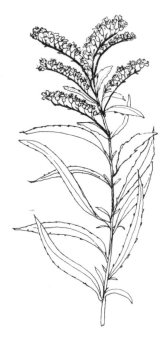

GOLDENROD

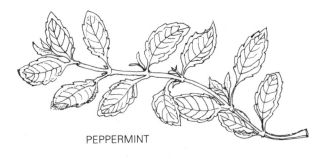

PEPPERMINT

55

Apple cider vinegar	Add 500 ml to your bathwater or apply full strength to the itchy spot.
Lemons	Apply fresh lemon juice directly onto the spot to ease irritation.
Oatmeal	Make a paste and moisten with elder tea (standard brew). Dab onto itchy area.
Elder	Wash with a strong brew of elder leaves. *Mint* leaves are also effective.

JAUNDICE

Include the following in the diet: asparagus (and drink the water in which it was cooked), oats, rye, sprouted wheat and wheatgrass, parsley, barley water and cooked barley grains.

Make a standard brew tea using either *Hypericum* flowers, *Asparagus*, *Parsley*, *Rosemary* or *Elder* flowers.

JOINTS, PAINFUL

Include the following in the diet: broccoli, Brussels sprouts, cauliflower, horseradish, grapefruit, guavas, lemons, oranges, parsley, green peppers, spinach, tomatoes, turnips and watercress.

Apple cider vinegar	Dip a clean cloth into the vinegar and apply, as hot as possible, to aching joints.
Castor oil plant	Warm a leaf and bind it over the painful joint. A *Cabbage* leaf will do as well.

Onion	Cut up a roasted onion and apply, as hot as can be tolerated, to the area. Bind in place.
Eucalyptus	Place leaves in a large pot (about 3 ℓ size), cover with water and boil up for 10 minutes. Strain, then add to bath-water. Add 500 ml *Epsom salts*.

See also FAVOURITE RECIPE 5: Herb tea for pain and inflammation.

KIDNEY AILMENTS

Include the following in the diet: fresh asparagus (drink the water in which it was cooked), radishes, melons (especially watermelon), pawpaw, summer squash, strawberries, watercress, fresh grated beetroot, avocado, cabbage, celery, dandelion greens, grapes and mangoes.

Make a standard brew tea using either *Parsley, Celery, Borage, Lucerne* or *Nettle*. Drink 125-250 ml at frequent intervals throughout the day (ie up to 6 cups).

Cayenne pepper	Include in the diet and add a pinch to herb teas.

LIVER COMPLAINTS

Include the following in the diet: apples, fresh grated raw beetroot, watercress, nasturtium, spring onions, peaches, pomegranates, asparagus, cabbage, broccoli, cauliflower, sweetcorn, cucumbers, dates, gooseberries, lettuce, lemons, quince, potatoes, raisins, sesame seeds, spinach, strawberries, tomatoes, walnuts and turnips.

Make a standard brew tea using either *Borage, Celery, Net-*

tle, Parsley, Comfrey, Burdock, Dandelion, Peppermint or *Rosemary*. They will give rapid relief, particularly after intake of drugs, alcohol or too-rich foods, on those 'off' days, by cleansing and stimulating a sluggish liver.

See also FAVOURITE RECIPE 8: Liver and gallbladder tonic.

MENOPAUSE see FAVOURITE RECIPE 10: Herb tea for menopause.

MENSTRUATION

Include the following in the diet if you are prone to heavy periods: carrots, lentils, cayenne pepper, cinnamon, lemon juice, parsley and ginger. Make a standard brew tea using either *Yarrow*, *Thyme* or *Raspberry* leaves. Drink 500 ml prior to and during menstruation.

If you have irregular, sparse menstruation, include the following in the diet: fresh grated beetroot, barley, green beans, strawberries, lettuce, brown rice and soya beans. Make a standard brew tea using either *Lemon balm* (melissa), *Fennel*, *Calendula*, *Basil*, *Dill* or *Nettle*.

To ease period pain any of the following herb teas will bring relief: *Feverfew*, *Chamomile*, *Catnip*, *Peppermint* or *Strawberry* leaves. Drink 3-5 cups per day before your period is due, and then during the first two days. Sweeten with honey if necessary.

NAUSEA

Sweet basil	Make a standard brew tea to ease symptoms. Sip with a squeeze of lemon juice. Teas made from *Peppermint*, *Mint* and *Bergamot* will do as well. Add a pinch of dried ginger.
Ginger	Place a small piece of root in a saucepan. Pour over 250 ml boiling water. Stand, steep, cool,

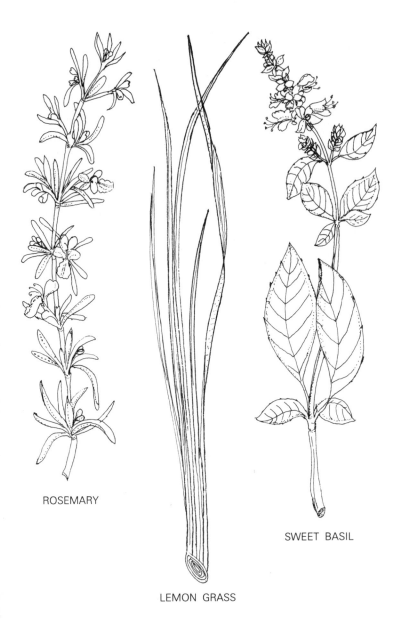

ROSEMARY

LEMON GRASS

SWEET BASIL

59

then strain. Sip slowly to relieve nausea.

Lemon   Squeeze a lemon into a glass of iced water. Add chips of ice. Sip frequently to relieve nausea.

NERVOUS TENSION (see also STRESS, IRRITABILITY and SEDATIVE)

Include the following in the diet: sunflower seeds, almonds, avocado, barley, beetroot, cabbage, maize oil, cherries, sweetcorn, dandelion greens, prunes, raisins, sesame seeds, dates, lettuce, mushrooms, peas, potatoes, brown rice, wheatgerm, spinach, walnuts, soya beans, tomatoes, turnips and nasturtium leaves.

Make a standard brew tea using either *Lemon balm* (melissa), *Catnip*, *Elderflowers*, *Feverfew*, *Marjoram*, *Lavender*, *Scented geranium*, *Chamomile*, *Celery* or *Rosemary*. Drink daily to calm nerves. Add 4-6 cloves for extra flavour. These teas will also soothe and relieve irritability.

See also FAVOURITE RECIPE 24: Exam-time tonic.

NEURALGIA (see also SEDATIVE)

For localised pain apply poultices of any of the following:

Allspice   Boil 250 ml berries in 500 ml boiling water. Crush to a paste and spread on a piece of gauze. Apply to the area and keep warm for 10 minutes.

Chamomile   Place hot teabags of chamomile tea against the painful area and keep covered. Replace from time to time with fresh hot teabags.

Horseradish Grate and scrape the root. Place on gauze, apply to the painful area and keep warm.

Lemon	Cut wedges of lemon and rub onto the painful area.
Peppermint	Warm leaves in hot water, apply to the area and cover with hot towels. Hold in place for 10 minutes.
Celery	Drink a standard brew tea during the day for relief of pain. *Sage* or *Catnip* tea will also be effective.

NIGHTMARES see FAVOURITE RECIPE 22: Herb tea for shock.

NIPPLES see BREASTS

NOSEBLEED

Yarrow Gently insert a wad of rolled up leaf into the nostril. Alternatively, drink a standard brew yarrow tea to stop the bleeding.

OBESITY (see also SLIMMING)

Include the following in the diet: apples, artichokes, fresh grated beetroot, broccoli, cabbage, fennel, melons (particularly watermelon), carrots, cauliflower, garlic, chives, endive, gooseberries, passion fruit, grapefruit, guavas, kumquats, lemons, oranges, lettuce, cucumber, loquats, nectarines, onions, okra, sweet peppers, pineapple, pomegranates, radishes, rhubarb, summer squash, tomatoes, turnips, watercress, nasturtium leaves, spring onions, apple cider vinegar, sunflower seeds, wheatgerm and plain yoghurt.

Make a standard brew tea using either *Fennel*, *Celery* or *Parsley*, or a combination of these herbs. Drink at least 3 times daily.

See also FAVOURITE RECIPE 9: Slimmer's tonic.

PAIN see ACHES AND STRAINS

PNEUMONIA

Include the following in the diet: figs, okra, onions, comfrey, garlic, mustard, lettuce, lucerne, barley sprouts, sunflower seeds, sweet potatoes, prunes, almonds, carrots and cabbage. Make vegetable broths using grated vegetables and barley.
Make a standard brew tea using *Comfrey, Violets* (leaves and flowers), *Maidenhair fern, Yarrow, Verbascum* (mullein), *Thyme* or *Winter savory*. Drink daily to regain strength.

POST-OPERATIVE TREATMENT

Include the following in the diet: barley drinks and soups (eat the cooked grain as a vegetable too), grapes, parsley, carrots, fresh grated beetroot, apples, apricots, dandelion greens, comfrey (chopped in soups).
   Make a standard brew tea using either *Comfrey, Sage* or *Salad burnet.*

Castor oil plant   Massage warm oil (or *Wheatgerm* oil) into scar *after the stitches have been removed.*

Vitamins   Add vitamins to your diet on your doctor's recommendation.

See also FAVOURITE RECIPE 23: Tonic wine.

PSORIASIS see FAVOURITE RECIPE 27: Problem skin tea.

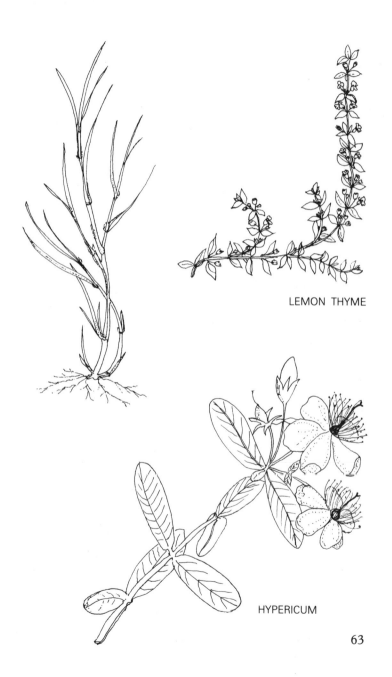

LEMON THYME

HYPERICUM

63

Make a wash or lotion of any of the following herbs: *Ajuga* (carpet bugle), *Aloe*, *Elder* (flowers and leaves), *Cornflowers*, *Honeysuckle* (flowers and leaves), *Soapwort* (flowers and leaves), *Parsley* or *Waterlily* (leaves and stems). Pick a potful and cover with water. Bring to the boil. Stand, steep and cool, then strain. Dab on frequently. Elderflowers and leaves and soapwort combine to make an excellent healing lotion.

RHEUMATISM

Include the following in the diet: artichokes, asparagus, melons, celery, fresh cherries, cucumbers, dandelion greens, garlic, figs, grapes, watermelon, kelp, lettuce, nectarines, oranges, strawberries, mandarins, watercress and chickweed.

Make a standard brew tea using either *Comfrey*, *Honeysuckle*, *Hypericum* flowers, *Nettle*, *Yarrow* or *Parsley*. Sip frequently.

See also FAVOURITE RECIPE 1: Rheumatism tea.

SEDATIVE

Make a standard brew tea using either *Lemon balm* (melissa), *Borage*, *Catnip*, *Elderflowers*, *Marjoram*, *Chamomile*, *Sage* or *Lavender*. Add 3-5 cloves to these teas. Drink before going to bed. The herbs can be combined according to taste, and sweetened with honey. Honey absorbs water, so it is helpful for water retention at night.

SHOCK see FAVOURITE RECIPE 22: Herb tea for shock.

SINUSITIS

Include the following in the diet: green salads, lucerne (alfal-

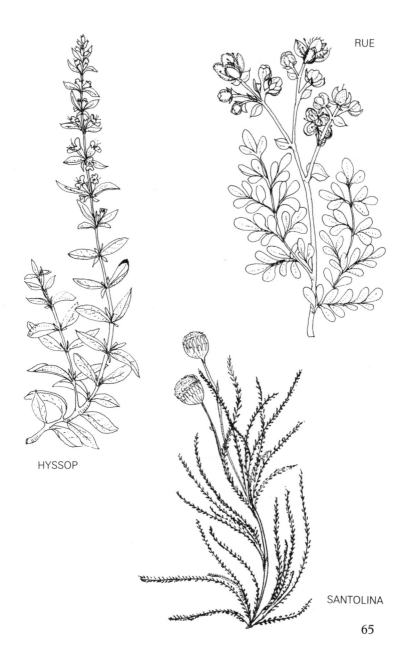

RUE

HYSSOP

SANTOLINA

65

fa) sprouts, comfrey, dandelion greens, salad burnet, carrots, lettuce, spinach, endive, sow's thistle, celery and parsley.

For sinusitis attacks drink a standard brew tea of either *Sage*, *Elderflowers*, *Peppermint* or *Spearmint*. To use as an inhalant, make a stronger brew, using just enough water to cover the herb. Bring to the boil and remove from the stove. Make a towel tent and inhale the fumes. Include a few drops of Olbas with the herbs. *Eucalyptus* leaves, *Rosemary* and *Pennyroyal* are all effective too. Use the cooled brew in the bath.

See also FAVOURITE RECIPE 25: Hayfever tea.

SKIN DISORDERS (see also ACNE)

Include the following in the diet: apples, beetroot tops, melons, rhubarb, broccoli, cabbage, carrots, cauliflower, coconuts (milk and flesh), dandelion greens, sow's thistle, figs, grapefruit, grapes, lemons, lettuce, pawpaw, peaches, pears, prunes, mandarins, salad burnet, watercress, nasturtium leaves and comfrey leaves. (Eat as much raw as possible.)

See also FAVOURITE RECIPE 27: Problem skin tea.

SLIMMING (see also OBESITY)

Include the following in the diet: asparagus, garlic, parsley, apple cider vinegar, sunflower seeds, apples, fresh grated beetroot, watermelon, carrots (including leaves), grapefruit, sliced fennel root, lemons, lettuce, loquats, green peppers, okra, summer squash, spinach, watercress, tomatoes and pomegranates.

Make a standard brew tea using *Celery*, *Parsley* or *Fennel* and drink daily.

See also FAVOURITE RECIPE 9: Slimmer's tonic.

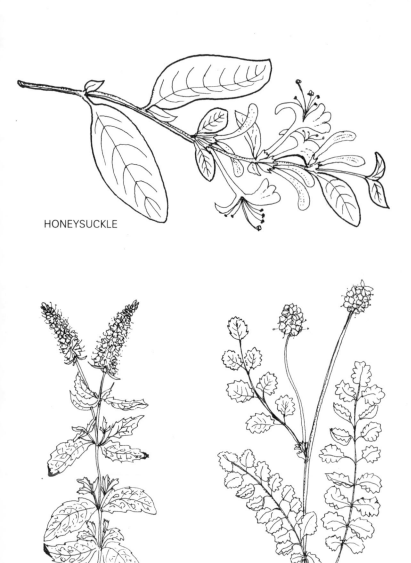

HONEYSUCKLE

MINT   SALAD BURNET

67

SORE THROAT (see also COLDS and COUGHS)

Make a standard brew tea using either *Yarrow, Bergamot, Elder flowers, Honeysuckle* flowers, *Rosemary, Sage, Thyme* or *Marjoram*. Drink twice daily to relieve symptoms.

Bergamot	Chop up and combine with lemon juice and honey to soothe the throat. Take 5 ml every hour.
Honey	Mix with lemon juice to ease the throat. Take 5 ml every now and then.
Apple cider vinegar	Dilute and gargle, swallowing a little as well.

See also FAVOURITE RECIPE 11: Elderflower gargle.

SPRAINS (see also ACHES AND STRAINS)

Onion	Warm slices of onion in hot water and apply to the area as a poultice. Sprigs of *Marjoram*, or a *Comfrey* or *Burdock* leaf can be used in the same way.
Mustard	Make a mustard plaster by crushing and pounding mustard seeds. Moisten with apple cider vinegar and apply on a strip of gauze to the area.
Apple cider vinegar	Dip a clean cloth into warmed vinegar, wring out and apply, as hot as possible, to the sprain. Change frequently.

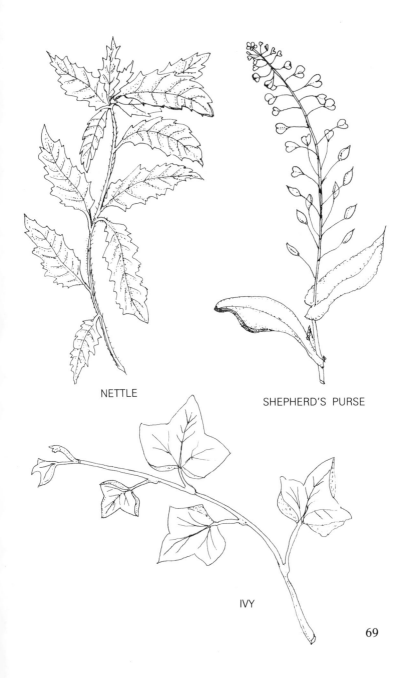

NETTLE

SHEPHERD'S PURSE

IVY

69

Include the following in the diet: grated apples and small pieces of crab-apple.

For stomachache and cramp, make a standard brew tea using either *Peppermint*, *Chamomile*, *Spearmint*, *Lemon balm* (melissa), *Lemon verbena*, *Fennel* (seeds too) or *Parsley*.

Ginger	Place a small piece of root in 250 ml boiling water. Stand and steep, then cool. Sip frequently to relieve pain.
Anise	Place a few aniseeds in 250 ml boiling water. Allow to cool. Sip frequently.
Cloves	Boil up 6 cloves in 250 ml water. Allow to cool, then sip frequently.
Cinnamon	Place half a cinnamon stick in 250 ml boiling water. Allow to cool, then sip frequently to bring relief.

See also FAVOURITE RECIPE 7: Herb tea for stomachache.

STRESS (see also IRRITABILITY, NERVOUS TENSION AND SEDATIVE)

Include the following in the diet: B vitamins, yoghurt, wheatgerm, borage, sunflower seeds, bran, Brewer's yeast, green vegetables, peaches, tomatoes, passion fruit, oats and oatmeal, and dandelion greens.

Standard brew teas of any of the following herbs will have a soothing, calming effect: *Lucerne*, *Comfrey*, *Lemon balm* (melissa), *Scented geranium*, red *Rose* petals, *Lavender*, *Sage*, *Chamomile*, *Catnip*, *Elderflowers*, *Lemon thyme* or *Rosemary*. Sweeten with honey if desired.

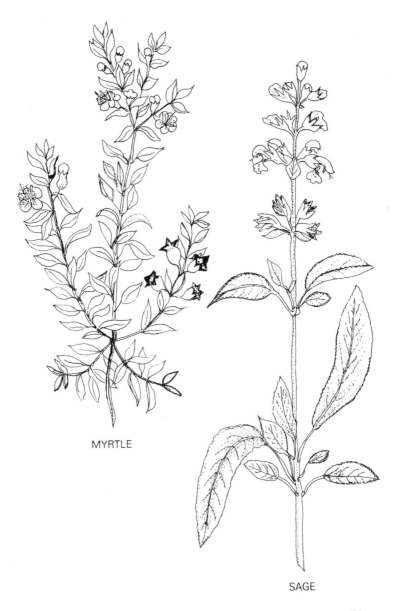

MYRTLE

SAGE

71

See also favourite recipe 23: Tonic wine.

sunburn

Drink plenty of fluids and herb teas (eg *Rosemary, Lemon grass*).

Aloe   Apply the juice of the leaf (*A. davyana* is excellent) to soothe the sunburn. *Waterlily* leaves (and stems) will also give relief.

Ajuga   Make a tea by boiling a potful of herbs with enough water to cover. Boil for 5 minutes. Stand, steep, cool. Strain and use as a wash. Alternatively, put into a bottle with a nozzle spray and spray the painful area every few minutes until it cools. *Salad burnet* and *Mint* can be used in the same way.

Milk   Dab onto the sunburnt area. *Yoghurt* is also effective.

Sow's thistle   Dab the milk onto a sunburnt nose for speedy relief.

Cucumber   Apply thin slices to painful areas.

swelling

Make packs of any of the following herbs and apply directly to the swollen area: *Parsley*, grated *Carrot, Castor oil* leaves, or leaves of *Lavender, Comfrey, Cabbage, Borage* or *Foxglove*. Warm the leaves first in hot water and apply hot to the area. Bind in place.

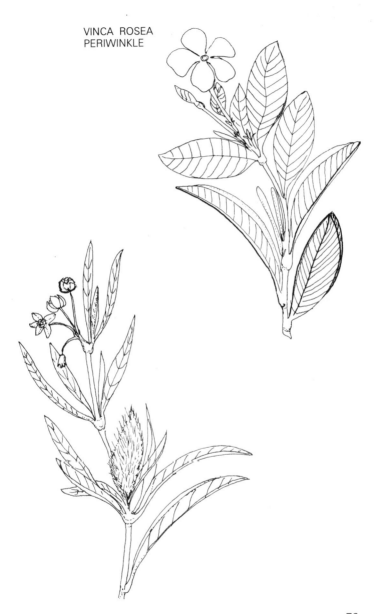

VINCA ROSEA
PERIWINKLE

73

Lavender   Dip a clean cloth in a strong tea (*Parsley* or
                Comfrey tea are also excellent) and dab the
                swollen area.

Witch hazel   If you can obtain the old-fashioned pure kind,
                it will quickly reduce puffiness and swelling (eg
                beneath the eyes) if dabbed on every now and
                then.

TAPEWORM see WORMS

TIREDNESS, LISTLESSNESS

Include the following in the diet: sprouts (very important,
especially mung beans and alfalfa), apricots, dried beans, lentils, fresh grated beetroot, Brazil nuts, broccoli, carrots, cauliflower, cabbage, sweetcorn, sesame seeds, sunflower seeds,
guavas, horseradish, lemons, lettuce, mustard greens, oranges,
parsley, peaches, pecan nuts, green peppers, sweet potatoes,
honey, soya beans, spinach, tomatoes and watercress.

Energy-giving teas can be made from *Rosemary* or *Lucerne*
(alfalfa). Use standard brew.

See also FAVOURITE RECIPE 14: Herb tea energiser, and 17:
Winter punch.

TONIC HERBS

Tonic herbs are needed to bring the body to peak health, particularly during a period of stress or anxiety, after an illness or
after over-indulgence of any kind. These herbs tone the whole
body from the inner blood tissues to the muscles, from the
inner organs to the skin.

Include the following in the diet: carrots and carrot juice,
cayenne pepper (add a pinch to teas and food), sprouts (par-

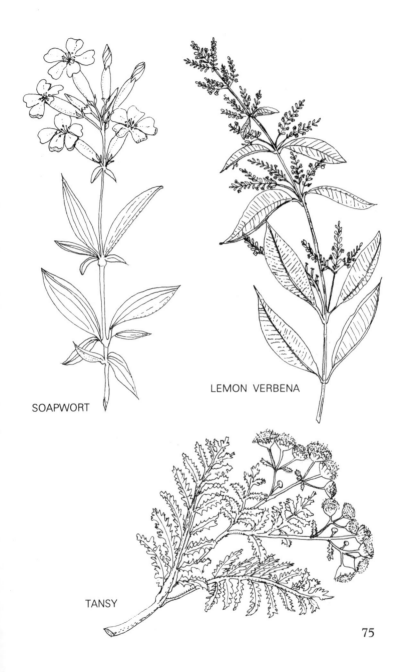

SOAPWORT

LEMON VERBENA

TANSY

75

ticularly alfalfa), sunflower seeds, watercress, dandelion greens and sesame seeds.

Make a standard brew tea using *Rosemary*, *Strawberry* leaves (eat the fruit), *Calendula* leaves and flowers, *Catnip*, *Chamomile*, *Chervil*, *Chicory*, *Goldenrod*, *Lucerne*, *Basil* or *Peppermint*.

Anise Bruise a few seeds, pour over 250 ml boiling water, then stand, steep and strain. Add lemon juice and honey and sip frequently. This is a powerful tonic.

TOOTHACHE

Make sure you visit your dentist regularly. If you have an aching tooth before you can get to him or her, chew a *Clove* or a wad of *Tarragon*. A little *Castor oil* dabbed onto the gum will also help.

To ensure strong enamel on the teeth, particularly in children, and to help prevent dental caries, include the following in the diet: apples, apricots, asparagus, green beans, fresh grated raw beetroot, carrots, broccoli, cabbage, melons, sweetcorn, dandelion greens, lettuce, oranges, pawpaw, parsley, borage, peaches, green peas, almonds, sunflower seeds, pecan nuts, sweet potatoes, prunes, spinach, watercress, comfrey and sow's thistle. Avoid sugars, starches and carbonated drinks. Use small amounts of honey as a sweetener.

ULCERS

Include the following in the diet: bland foods such as brown rice, oatmeal, steamed vegetables, pawpaw, steamed apples and steamed comfrey leaves.

Make a standard brew tea using *Comfrey*, *Chamomile*, *Scented geranium* or *Lavender*.

Comfrey	Pulp root and leaf and apply to the area. Use a fresh poultice daily.
Periwinkle	Use *Vinca major* and make a strong tea (250 ml leaves and flowers to 250 ml boiling water) and apply daily as a lotion or use as a wash. Dab on frequently.
Aloe	Apply the leaf jelly to the area.
Potato	For stomach ulcers eat a small piece of raw potato (walnut sized) before a meal. It will take the pain away and heal the ulcer.

VARICOSE VEINS

Include the following in the diet: plenty of fresh fruit and vegetables, and water.

Make a standard brew tea using *Lemon balm*, *Lemon grass* or *Lemon thyme*, adding honey to sweeten.

Calendula	Make a strong tea (250 ml herb to 500 ml boiling water). Stand, steep, then strain. Use as a lotion or wash. Apply while still hot, either dabbed onto the area or as a poultice. Dip a cloth into the tea, wring out and apply. Cover with a piece of plastic and bind in place. Replace with further hot applications until the area feels better. *Tansy* and *Oak* leaves are also good used this way.
	Calendula petals can also be used to make a standard brew tea. Drink daily. Add cayenne pepper to every drink during the day, starting with a pinch and working up to $\frac{1}{8}$th of a teaspoon per day.

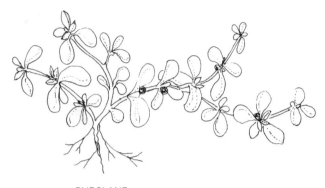

PURSLANE

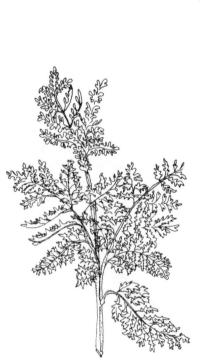

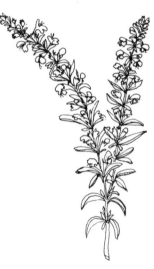

WINTER SAVORY

78

Mint   To ease vomiting, take frequent sips of a strong tea –
125 ml herb to 250 ml boiling water. Stand, steep,
strain. Sip while hot.

WARTS

Apply any of the following directly onto the wart, at regular
intervals: juice of a *Fig* leaf, *Apple* juice squeezed from a fresh,
sour apple, *Cabbage* leaf juice, *Dandelion* leaf milk, *Sow's thistle*
milk, fresh *Pineapple* juice, *Watercress* juice or juice from the
purple *Wandering Jew* (purple tradescantia).

Tradescantia   Bind a piece of tradescantia in place over
the wart. Use a fresh piece every day.

Banana   Take a small piece of skin and place it,
inside down, over the wart. Bind in
place. Repeat daily for 10 days.

Pig's ear cotyledon   Slightly crush and bind in place. Repeat
daily for 10 days. (This is excellent for
plantar warts.)

Wheatgerm   Apply oil frequently to the wart.

WORMS

Include the following in the diet: apples, onions, garlic, green
pepper, peaches, pineapple, pomegranate, sesame seeds, nasturtium seeds, sweet basil and rhubarb.

Carrots   125-250 ml grated raw carrots and 3 cloves garlic eaten first thing in the morning will help expel worms.

Garlic	Eat a whole peeled clove first thing in the morning.
Horseradish	Grate fresh root. Spread 1 dessertspoon on a little brown bread and eat first thing in the morning.
Lemons	Drink freshly squeezed juice (125 ml with a little hot water) first thing in the morning. Sip frequently throughout the day.
Pumpkin	Eat 7 pips as soon as you get up in the morning (ie on an empty stomach) every day for 10 days. Chew well.
Tansy	Eat a teaspoon of seeds on an empty stomach.
Thyme	Eat 2 fresh sprigs and drink 250 ml standard brew thyme tea on an empty stomach.

WOUNDS

Include the following in the diet: comfrey, nasturtium leaves, violets (leaves and flowers) and apples.

Make a strong brew tea using 500 ml herb boiled up in 750 ml water for 3 minutes. Stand, steep, strain. Use warm to wash the wound or to soak a dressing. Any of these herbs will be effective: *Bergamot, Thyme, Calendula* (petals and leaves),

Comfrey, *Cornflowers*, *Grape* leaves and tendrils, *Hypericum*, *Hollyhock*, *Nasturtium* or *Periwinkle* (Vinca major).

Comfrey   Use pounded comfrey as a dressing. *Calendula* petals and leaves can be used in the same way.

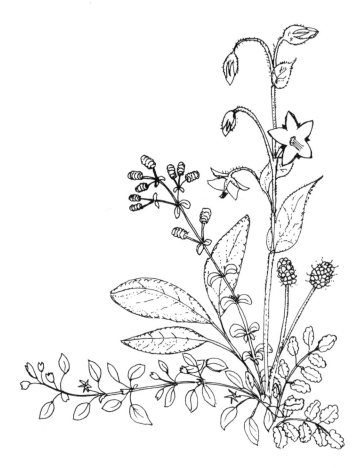

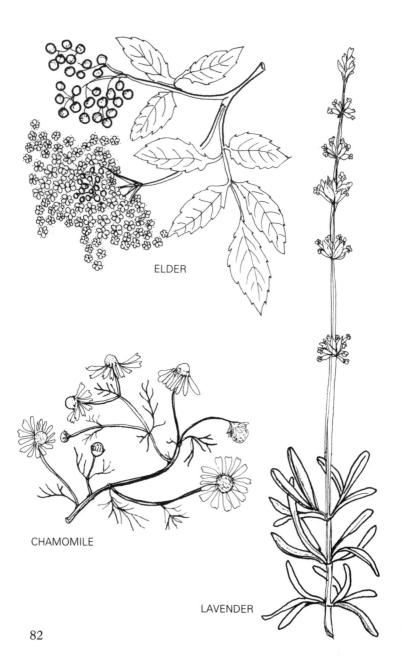

ELDER

CHAMOMILE

LAVENDER

82

Favourite Recipes for Common Ailments

The following are some of my personal favourite remedies, all of which have been tried and tested many times over. As I always use fresh herbs, these recipes are worked on fresh herb measurements.

1 RHEUMATISM TEA

37,5 ml celery seed
37,5 ml chopped nettle
37,5 ml elderflowers
37,5 ml yarrow
37,5 ml dandelion root
5 ml cayenne pepper

Boil herbs in 3 ℓ water for 5 minutes. Stand, steep, cool, then strain. Add cayenne pepper. Warm up and drink 2-3 cups of this brew each day. Keep excess in the fridge. Keep up treatment for 2 weeks. This is a wonderfully soothing and alkalising tea and it is as effective for GOUT as it is for rheumatism.

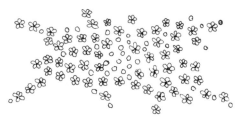

2 FEVER DRINK

500 ml elderflowers
500 ml peppermint leaves
250 ml yarrow leaves

Boil up in 2,5 ℓ water for 5 minutes. Stand, steep, strain. While still hot drink a cup of this brew and follow it immediately with a hot bath. Repeat every 4 hours. Bed rest is recommended until the fever subsides. This tea will minimise symptoms and, if taken immediately the symptoms start, will greatly hasten recovery.

3 HERB TEA FOR CRAMP

1 thumb-length piece ginger root
250 ml chamomile flowers
250 ml lemon balm leaves
250 ml hypericum flowers

Boil herbs in 3 ℓ water for 5-10 minutes, keeping pot covered. Stand, steep, strain. Add a pinch of cayenne and drink 250 ml during the attack and then daily for 3-6 days. Keep excess in the fridge.

4 HEADACHE TEA

12,5 ml rosemary
12,5 ml lavender
12,5 ml lemon balm
12,5 ml peppermint
750 ml water

Bring water and herbs to the boil, and then immediately remove from stove and leave to cool. Drink 125 ml every hour for 3-4 hours to ease headache pain.

5 HERB TEA FOR PAIN AND INFLAMMATION

37,5 ml comfrey leaves and root
small piece ginger root
37,5 ml calendula flowers
25 ml verbascum flowers
25 ml hypericum flowers
25 ml plantain leaves

Blend herbs together in a grinder. Add a little castor oil and apply to the painful area on a piece of clean gauze.

6 ANAEMIA SOUP

250 ml chives
500 ml stinging nettle
500 ml salad burnet
250 ml dandelion root and leaves
250 ml lucerne leaves

Chop herbs finely. Blend together to make into a soup, adding a little Marmite or soy sauce with the water. Boil for 5 minutes and drink a cup or two daily.

7 HERB TEA FOR STOMACHACHE

125 ml peppermint leaves
12,5 ml fennel seeds and leaves
250 ml lemon balm leaves
1 piece ginger root

Boil herbs in just over 1 ℓ water for 5 minutes. Stand and steep. Take 125 ml every 15 minutes until the condition clears. This tea is also good for FLATULENCE.

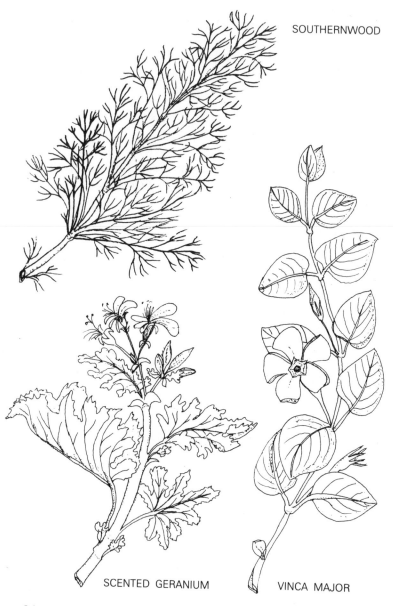

SOUTHERNWOOD

SCENTED GERANIUM

VINCA MAJOR

86

8 LIVER AND GALLBLADDER TONIC

250 ml lemon balm leaves
25 ml parsley root and stems
125 ml dandelion roots
750 ml water

Boil herbs together in water and immediately remove from stove. Stand, steep and cool. Sip 125 ml at intervals throughout the day.

9 SLIMMER'S TONIC

250 ml chickweed
3 cinnamon sticks
750 ml dandelion leaves and roots
750 ml fennel leaves, stems and seeds

Bring to the boil in 2,5 ℓ water. Stand, steep, strain. Drink 125-250 ml 3 times a day before meals.

10 HERB TEA FOR MENOPAUSE

500 ml raspberry leaves
125 ml parsley stems and root
500 ml lemon balm leaves
250 ml goldenrod leaves and flowers
250 ml hypericum flowers

Boil herbs together in 3 ℓ water for 3 minutes. Stand, steep, cool, then strain. Drink 250 ml daily. This tea eases flushes and stress, as well as fluid retention.

11 ELDERFLOWER GARGLE

This is an excellent brew for sore throats and coughs.

250 ml fresh elderflowers, or 125 ml dried
250 ml sage leaves
750 ml water
10 ml almond oil
25 ml honey
10 cloves

Boil herbs and water for 3 minutes. Stand, steep, strain. Add oil and honey. Keep in a screwtop bottle. Warm up before gargling. Use frequently.

12 WINTER WARM TONIC

1 bottle sherry
2 sticks cinnamon
10 cloves
pinch or two cayenne pepper
250 ml sage leaves
27,5 ml honey

Add the herbs, spices and honey to the sherry. Shake up the bottle. Store for 1 month, shaking daily. Drink a small sherry glassful on winter evenings, especially when you come in chilled. This is an excellent method of warding off coughs and colds.

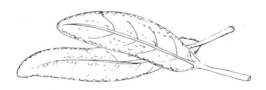

13 POOR CIRCULATION HERB DRINK

2 cinnamon sticks
10 cloves
1 thumb-length piece ginger
2-5 ml cayenne pepper
125 ml dandelion roots
250 ml chopped, cleaned rose-hips
25 ml honey
37,5 ml brandy

Boil herbs and spices together in 1 ℓ water. Stand, steep, strain. Add honey and brandy. Sip a sherry glass of this mixture 3 times a day. Step up dose during the winter.

14 HERB TEA ENERGISER

250 ml lucerne leaves
250 ml peppermint or spearmint
125 ml rosemary
honey
lemon juice

Place herbs in a pot and pour over 1,5 ℓ boiling water. Stand, steep, strain. Add honey and lemon to taste. Drink a cup, either hot or iced, at intervals throughout the day to combat tiredness and listlessness.

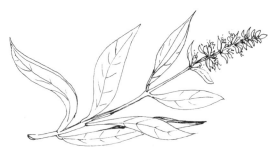

15 HERB TEA DIGESTIVE AID

125 ml peppermint leaves
250 ml lemon balm leaves
125 ml lemon verbena leaves

Place herbs in a pot and pour over 1,5 ℓ boiling water. Stand, steep, strain. Add honey and lemon to taste. Drink after a heavy meal or in the event of a heartburn attack.

16 HERB TEA SLEEP AID

12,5 ml lavender
12,5 ml lemon balm
12,5 ml red rose petals
honey

Place herbs in a pot and pour over 250-500 ml boiling water. Stand, steep, strain. Sweeten with honey. Drink warm last thing at night.

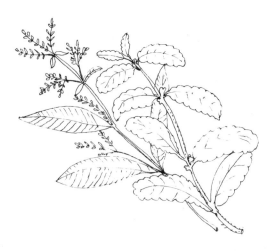

17 WINTER PUNCH

4 Granny Smith apples, sliced
2 lemons
125 ml rosemary twigs
1,5 ℓ water
25 ml apple cider vinegar
few raisins
50 ml honey
6 cloves

Boil up apples, add juice of lemons, water, cloves, raisins and rosemary. Simmer for 10 minutes. Stand and steep. Strain through a sieve. Pour into mugs. Add honey and apple cider vinegar and the raisins from the sieve. Sip while hot. After a hard day this drink will revitalise flagging energy and spirits.

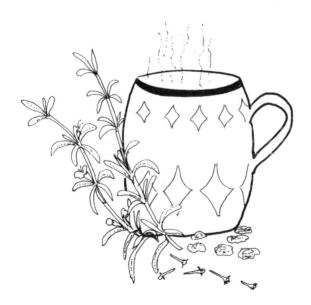

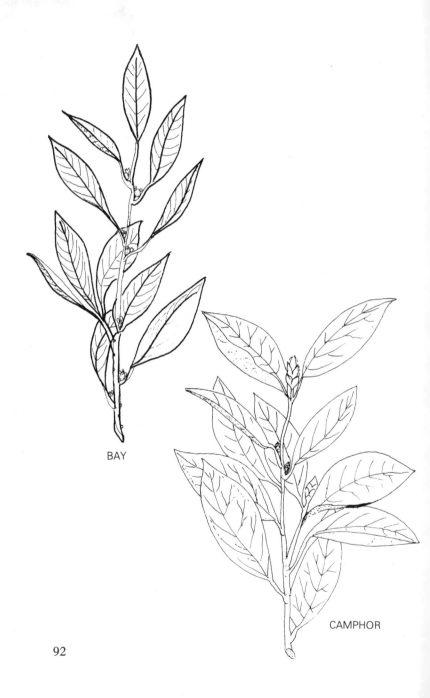

BAY

CAMPHOR

18 VINEGAR OF THE FOUR THIEVES

This vinegar has a fascinating legend. During the time of the bubonic plague, four notorious thieves continuously ransacked plague-ridden houses. They were finally caught and brought before a judge in a court in Marseilles. When asked how they managed to keep healthy and free of contamination in those plague-ridden houses, they offered their secret recipe in return for their freedom. Their request was granted and this is the recipe:

2 ℓ apple cider vinegar
25 ml fresh lavender leaves and flowers
25 ml rosemary
25 ml sage
25 ml rue
25 ml garlic cloves, peeled
25 ml wormwood
25 ml mint

Combine all the herbs except the garlic. Steep in the vinegar and stand in the sun for 2 weeks. Strain and bottle. Add the garlic cloves and leave for another week. Strain. Keep in the fridge. Take 5 ml frequently throughout the day to ward off winter flu (this is best done in early autumn). During an epidemic use it to wash walls and floors in the sickroom; wash with it, and wash the patient in it too.

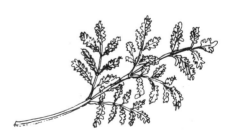

19 HERBAL MASSAGE OIL

This is an excellent, deeply penetrating oil for tired muscles. I use it on aching feet after a long hike; it is also very relaxing for aching backs and necks.

500 ml sweet oil
12,5 ml hydrous lanolin
12,5 ml wheatgerm oil
12,5 ml dried lavender flowers
12,5 ml dried rosemary
12,5 ml dried scented geranium leaves
12,5 ml calendula flowers

Blend the oils. Steep the dried herbs in a bottle containing the oils. Shake well daily. Keep out of direct sunlight, but keep in a warm place for 3 weeks. Strain out the herbs, pressing out all the oil. Pour into clean jars and store in a cool dark place. The secret is to massage the oil deeply into the tired area, and then to soak in a hot bath. You may also add a strong rosemary brew to the bathwater.

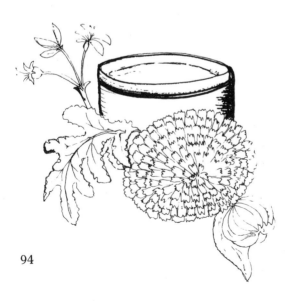

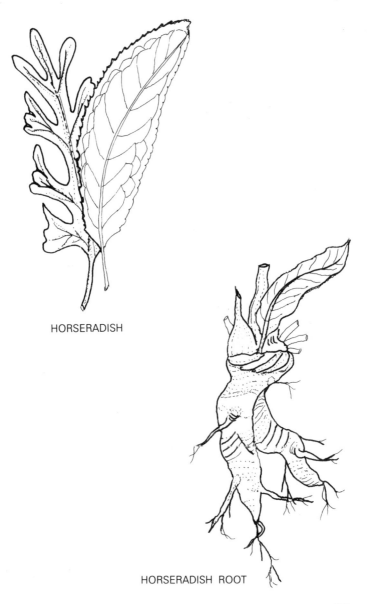

HORSERADISH

HORSERADISH ROOT

95

20 HIKER'S ENERGY BALLS

When you feel yourself starting to flag, instead of a bar of chocolate, pop one of these energy balls into your mouth to give you a lift and put new spring in your step.

500 ml each dried figs, dates and prunes
250 ml wheat sprouts
250 ml sesame seeds
250 ml sunflower seeds
12,5 ml honey
little water

Put the sunflower and sesame seeds through a coffee grinder. Roughly chop up fruit and put through a mincer or food grinder. Mix well, add honey and enough water to make a paste. Pinch off pieces and roll into balls. Roll into sesame seeds, coconut, wheatgerm etc. Wrap in greased paper and keep in the fridge. These are the best pick-me-ups for hikers and backpackers, but for the weary after a hard day in the office they also work wonders.

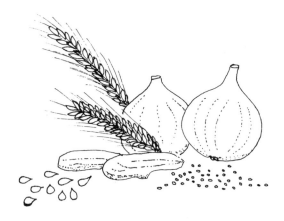

21 HERB DEODORANT

5 ml cloves
12,5 ml coriander seeds
5 ml cassia
25 ml lavender flowers, dried
10 ml dried thyme
25 ml dried sage

Grind up all the ingredients in a hand mill or grinder. Add to a cup of bland talcum powder (eg baby powder) and use to dust under arms etc.

22 HERB TEA FOR SHOCK

250 ml lemon balm leaves
125 ml lavender leaves and flowers
125 ml scented geranium leaves
125 ml chamomile flowers
125 ml comfrey leaves

Place herbs in a pot and pour over 1,5 ℓ boiling water. Stand, steep, strain. Sweeten with honey and drink warm (125 ml) every half hour to calm and soothe. Keep excess in the fridge and warm as required. It is effective for hysteria and night-mares.

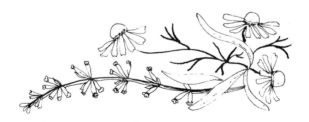

23 TONIC WINE

This tonic is beneficial to people under stress or for someone recovering from an illness.

1 bottle red wine
2 pieces rosemary (approx 15 cm long)
1 stick cinnamon
1 small piece ginger root
10 cloves
1 piece cleaned dandelion root (approx 15 cm long)

Steep all the ingredients in the wine for 2 weeks. Cork and keep in the fridge. Shake daily. Strain and drink a small wine-glass every evening.

24 EXAM-TIME TONIC

This excellent brew supplies minerals and vitamins in an easily assimilated form. For overtired students at exam time, it cannot be bettered.

500 ml lucerne leaves and flowers
250 ml chickweed
500 ml dandelion leaves
250 ml parsley leaves and stems
250 ml rosemary leaves
500 ml stinging nettle leaves
125 ml catnip leaves and flowers
125 ml yarrow leaves

Place herbs in a pot and pour over 4 ℓ boiling water. Stand, steep, cool, then strain. Add lemon juice and honey to taste and drink a cup warm 2 or 3 times a day. Keep excess in the fridge.

25 HAYFEVER TEA

500 ml sage leaves
250 ml elderflowers
250 ml peppermint leaves
250 ml lemon verbena

Place herbs in a pot and pour over 4 ℓ boiling water. Stand, steep, cool, then strain. Drink one cup, either hot or cold, sweetened with honey, first thing in the morning and again at midday. (Add a drop of Olbas to the tea if you like.) Keep excess in the fridge. Warm a little as you need it. During attacks, sip hot tea frequently. It is also effective for SINUSITIS.

26 HERB TEA FOR BRONCHITIS AND ASTHMA

250 ml verbascum flowers and leaves
250 ml violet flowers and leaves
250 ml comfrey flowers and leaves
250 ml lemon juice
250 ml lucerne leaves

Mix herbs together and pour over 2 ℓ boiling water. Stand, steep, cool, then strain. Sweeten with honey. Drink 125 ml frequently throughout the day. Store excess in the fridge. Warm a little as you need it.

I find this a wonderfully soothing tea which breaks that tight, chesty feeling. It clears mucus and lifts the cough.

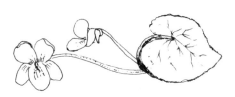

27 PROBLEM SKIN TEA

This tea is a skin cleanser; if taken daily, it will clear acne and pimples and tone the skin. Use any leftover tea as a face wash.

250 ml lemon balm leaves
250 ml mint leaves
250 ml dandelion leaves and root
125 ml parsley leaves and stems
500 ml burdock leaves and root
250 ml red clover flowers

Boil up ingredients in 3 ℓ water for 5 minutes. Stand, steep, cool, then strain. Drink 3 cups daily, at intervals, warm or cold. Add lemon juice and honey. This brew is also excellent for PSORIASIS and ECZEMA. Drink as above or dab onto the affected areas.

28 HERBAL MOUTHWASH

500 ml apple cider vinegar
250 ml water
10 cloves
250 ml rosemary leaves

Soak the rosemary and cloves in the apple cider vinegar for 24 hours. Add warm water. Shake well, strain and bottle. Keep on the bathroom shelf and use daily as a gargle and mouthwash.

29 CONSTIPATION REMEDY

Probably the most effective way of clearing up this problem, this recipe needs to be eaten every day with breakfast porridge, or pawpaw, yoghurt, muesli etc, until the bowel becomes regular.

20 ml bran (Digestive Bran – "Semels")
20 ml skim milk powder
20 ml sunflower oil

Mix together and add to porridge etc.

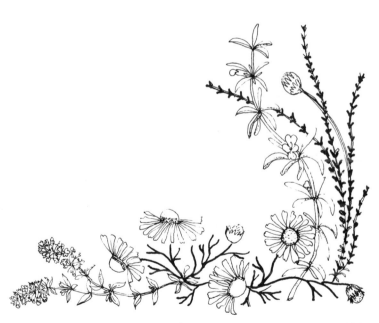

Notes

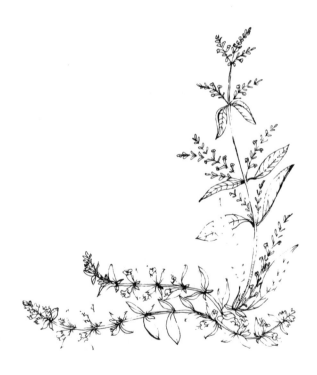

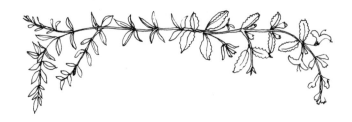

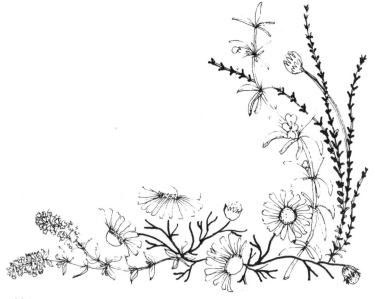

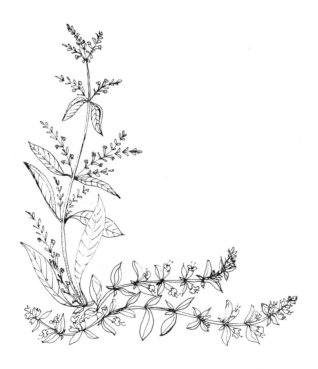

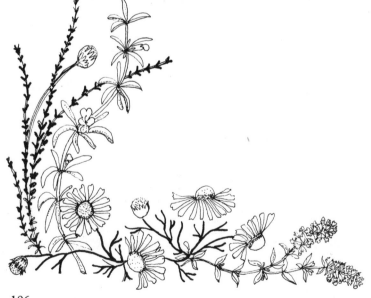